Chapter 1: Foundations of Nursing Pharmacology

1.1. Introduction to Phar

Pharmacology is the science of drugs—t
effects, and medical applications. Unders
healthcare professionals, especially nurses, as it ensures safe and
effective medication administration to patients.

The Three Core Concepts of Pharmacology

Pharmacology can be broken down into three fundamental areas:

- **Pharmacokinetics** – How the body absorbs, distributes, metabolizes, and eliminates drugs.
- **Pharmacodynamics** – How drugs interact with the body at the biochemical and physiological levels.
- **Pharmacotherapeutics** – The practical use of drugs to prevent or treat diseases.

Additionally, this chapter explores other key aspects, such as how drugs are named and classified, where they come from, how they are administered, and how new drugs are developed.

Understanding Drug Names and Classifications

Each drug has three different names:

- Chemical Name – A detailed scientific name based on its molecular composition.
- Generic Name – A simpler, standardized name derived from the chemical name.
- Trade Name – The brand name assigned by pharmaceutical companies, often trademarked (®).

To avoid confusion, healthcare professionals primarily use the generic name, as a single drug can have multiple trade names.

The Importance of Standardized Drug Naming

In 1962, the U.S. government mandated that each drug have a single official name, listed in the United States Pharmacopeia (USP) and National Formulary (NF) to ensure consistency and safety.

Drug Classification

Drugs are categorized based on their characteristics and effects:

- **Pharmacologic Class** – Grouped based on shared chemical properties or mechanisms of action (e.g., beta-blockers).
- **Therapeutic Class** – Grouped based on the conditions they treat (e.g., antihypertensives for high blood pressure).

Origins of Drugs: Where Do They Come From?

Traditionally, medications were derived from natural sources such as:

- **Plants** – Early medicine used various plant parts, though these could contain impurities.
- **Animals** – Some hormones and enzymes are extracted from animal sources.
- **Minerals** – Certain drugs are formulated using natural minerals like iron, iodine, and magnesium sulfate.

Today, most medications are synthetically developed in laboratories, allowing for higher purity, precision, and effectiveness.

Advancements in Drug Development

Scientific research has revolutionized pharmacology with synthetic drugs and genetic engineering. Techniques like recombinant DNA technology have enabled the production of essential medications, such as synthetic insulin, which was previously extracted from animal sources.

PHARMACOLOGY
DECODED

Essential Concepts Made Simple – For Students, Nurses

and Medical Beginners

Victoria Anderson

Table of Contents

Methods of Drug Administration

The method of administration affects how quickly and effectively a drug works. Common administration routes include:

- **Oral (PO)** – The most common and convenient method (e.g., tablets, capsules, syrups).
- **Intravenous (IV)** – Directly into the bloodstream for immediate effect.
- **Intramuscular (IM)** – Injected into the muscle for quick absorption.
- **Subcutaneous (SubQ)** – Injected just under the skin for slower absorption.
- **Topical** – Applied directly to the skin or mucous membranes.
- **Inhalation** – Breathed into the lungs for rapid action.
- **Rectal/Vaginal** – Suppositories, creams, or ointments for localized or systemic effects.
- Some specialized methods include epidural injections, intra-articular injections (into joints), and intrathecal injections (into the spinal canal).

Animal-Derived Medications

Some drugs originate from animal sources, utilizing body fluids or glands to create effective treatments. Examples include:

- **Hormones** – Insulin, extracted from animals in the past, is now mostly synthesized.
- **Oils and Fats** – Cod-liver oil is a well-known example, rich in essential nutrients.
- **Enzymes** – Substances like pancreatin and pepsin help with digestion.
- **Vaccines** – Created using killed, weakened, or modified microorganisms to boost immunity.

Minerals as Medicine

Certain metallic and nonmetallic minerals are essential in drug formulations, providing materials that can't be sourced from plants or animals. These minerals are used either in their natural form or combined with other compounds to enhance their effectiveness. Examples include:

- **Iron** – Essential for treating anemia.
- **Iodine** – A key ingredient in thyroid medications.
- **Epsom Salts (Magnesium Sulfate)** – Used for muscle relaxation and detoxification.

Laboratory Innovations: The Future of Medicine

Most modern medications are created in laboratories, allowing for better precision and fewer impurities than natural sources. Some notable examples include:

- **Thyroid Hormones** – Once derived from animals, now produced synthetically.
- **Cimetidine** – A synthetic drug used to treat acid reflux and ulcers.

The Role of DNA Research in Drug Development

Advancements in genetic engineering have revolutionized medicine. Scientists use recombinant DNA technology to develop genetically modified bacteria that can produce essential medications, such as synthetic insulin for diabetic patients.

Drug Administration: How Medications Enter the Body

The way a drug is administered affects how quickly and effectively it works. The route of administration determines the dosage, absorption speed, and patient response. Common Routes of Administration are:

Sublingual, Buccal, and Translingual Administration

Certain medications, like nitroglycerin, dissolve under the tongue (sublingual), inside the cheek (buccal), or on the tongue (translingual). These methods help the drug bypass digestion, allowing faster absorption into the bloodstream.

Gastric Administration

When patients can't take medications orally, drugs can be delivered directly into the gastrointestinal (GI) system through a tube, such as a gastric tube (G-tube).

Intradermal Administration

For diagnostic purposes, drugs are injected just below the skin's surface using a fine needle at a 10- to 15-degree angle. This is commonly used for allergy tests and tuberculosis screening.

Intramuscular (IM) Injections

IM injections deliver medication deep into the muscle, allowing for faster absorption and larger doses (up to 3 mL). This method is useful for drugs that can't be taken orally, such as certain vaccines and hormonal treatments.

Intravenous (IV) Administration

IV administration directly delivers drugs into the bloodstream, making it the fastest way to introduce medications into the body. This method is used for:

- Fluids (for hydration and electrolyte balance).
- Blood transfusions.
- Diagnostic contrast agents (for imaging tests).
- Emergency medications (such as pain relievers and antibiotics).

Oral (PO) Administration

The most common method, where pills, capsules, or liquids are taken by mouth. It is also the safest and most cost-effective option for medication delivery. However, it requires the patient to be conscious and able to swallow.

Rectal and Vaginal Administration

Some drugs are absorbed through the rectal or vaginal mucosa in the form of:

- **Suppositories** – Solid medications inserted into the rectum or vagina.
- **Ointments, creams, and gels** – Used for treating infections or local conditions.

Certain rectally administered drugs can also have systemic effects, meaning they enter the bloodstream to treat the entire body.

Respiratory Administration

Drugs that are in gas or mist form can be inhaled for rapid absorption. This method is commonly used for:

- Asthma inhalers (metered-dose inhalers).
- Nebulizers for breathing treatments.

Emergency drugs administered directly into the lungs via an endotracheal tube.

Subcutaneous (SubQ) Injections

A small dose of medication (up to 1 mL) is injected beneath the skin, typically in the upper arm, thigh, or abdomen. This method allows for gradual absorption and is commonly used for:

- Insulin injections for diabetes.
- Heparin to prevent blood clots.

Topical Administration

Medications can also be applied directly to the skin or mucous membranes, such as:

- Dermatologic creams for rashes or skin conditions.

- Eye drops (ophthalmic) for infections or dryness.
- Ear drops (otic) to treat ear infections.
- Nasal sprays for allergies or congestion.

Specialized Infusions: Targeted Drug Delivery

Some drugs are administered directly to a specific body site through specialized infusions. These include:

- **Epidural** – Injected into the epidural space near the spine, commonly used for pain relief during labor.
- **Intrapleural** – Delivered into the pleural cavity (lungs) to treat conditions like pleural effusion.
- **Intraperitoneal** – Injected into the abdominal cavity, often for chemotherapy.
- **Intraosseous** – Delivered into the bone marrow, used in emergency situations when IV access is difficult.
- **Intra-articular** – Injected into joints to treat arthritis or inflammation.
- **Intrathecal** – Injected directly into the spinal canal, often used for pain management or chemotherapy.

The Drug Development Process

In the past, discovering new drugs was based largely on trial and error. Today, drug development follows a structured scientific process monitored by the FDA (Food and Drug Administration).

How New Drugs Are Approved

Before a drug can be sold, researchers must conduct extensive animal studies and clinical trials to assess its safety and effectiveness. Only after a rigorous review does the FDA approve an application for an Investigational New Drug (IND).

Fast-Tracked Drug Approvals

Under certain conditions, the FDA can expedite drug approval. For example, due to the HIV/AIDS crisis, the FDA introduced a fast-track process to speed up the availability of life-saving drugs.

If a drug reaches Phase II or III clinical trials, its sponsor can apply for Treatment IND status.

Once approved, the drug can be distributed to doctors for use in patients who meet the eligibility criteria.

Fast-tracked drugs are closely monitored to ensure safety and effectiveness, even after approval.

1.2. Pharmacokinetics

Pharmacokinetics is the study of how drugs travel through the body from the moment they are taken to the moment they are eliminated. This process involves four key stages:

- **Absorption** – How the drug enters the bloodstream.
- **Distribution** – How it spreads to different tissues and organs.
- **Metabolism** – How the body processes the drug for elimination.
- **Excretion** – How the drug leaves the body.

Pharmacokinetics also helps determine when a drug starts working (onset of action), when it reaches its highest concentration in the body (peak level), and how long it remains effective (duration of action).

Absorption: Getting the Drug into the Body

Absorption refers to how a drug moves from the site of administration into the bloodstream. The speed and efficiency of absorption depend on several factors, including the route of administration, blood flow, and the drug's formulation.

How Drugs Are Absorbed

At a cellular level, drugs enter the body through two main processes:

Passive Transport (No Energy Required)

The drug moves naturally from an area of higher concentration to an area of lower concentration (diffusion).

This process requires no energy and happens with small molecules that can easily pass through cell membranes.

Most oral medications use this method, moving from the digestive tract into the bloodstream.

Active Transport (Energy Required)

The body actively moves the drug from an area of lower concentration to an area of higher concentration.

This process requires energy and is used to absorb important substances like electrolytes (sodium, potassium) and specific drugs (levodopa for Parkinson's disease).

Pinocytosis (Cell Drinking)

In this unique form of active transport, cells engulf the drug particles and pull them inside.

This process is mainly used for absorbing fat-soluble vitamins (A, D, E, and K).

Factors affecting absorption

Several factors influence how fast and efficiently a drug is absorbed:

Fast-Absorbing Drugs

Drugs that directly enter the bloodstream (e.g., IV injections) or dissolve quickly (e.g., sublingual tablets) are absorbed almost immediately.

Examples: Nitroglycerin (under the tongue), inhaled asthma medications, and IV pain relievers.

Moderate-Absorbing Drugs

Medications taken orally, injected into muscles (IM), or injected under the skin (SubQ) take longer to absorb because they must pass through different membranes before reaching the bloodstream.

Examples: Antibiotics, insulin, and most vaccines.

Slow-Absorbing Drugs

Some medications are designed for gradual release and can take hours or even days to fully absorb.

Examples: Rectal suppositories, extended-release tablets, and transdermal patches (e.g., nicotine patches).

Additional Factors That Impact Absorption

If a patient has had part of their small intestine removed, absorption is reduced because there's less surface area for drug absorption.

Liver Function & First-Pass Effect

Drugs taken orally must pass through the liver before reaching circulation.

The liver breaks down a portion of the drug, sometimes reducing its strength before it reaches the bloodstream. This is known as the first-pass effect.

To compensate, some oral drugs require higher doses or are given through non-oral routes (like IV or sublingual).

Blood Flow & Absorption

More blood flow = faster absorption.

Example: Muscles with higher blood flow (like the deltoid in the arm) absorb drugs faster than areas with lower circulation (gluteal muscle in the buttocks).

Pain & Stress

Pain and stress can slow absorption because they reduce blood circulation and digestion speed.

Food & Drug Absorption

High-fat meals slow down stomach emptying, delaying drug absorption.

Some drugs work better when taken with food, while others are best taken on an empty stomach.

Drug Formulation & Coatings

Liquid medications absorb faster than tablets or capsules.

Enteric-coated drugs are designed to pass through the stomach and dissolve in the intestines to prevent irritation.

Drug Interactions

Some drugs interact with other medications or food, either increasing or decreasing absorption.

Distribution: How Drugs Travel in the Body

Once a drug is absorbed, it moves through the bloodstream to reach different tissues and organs. The rate and extent of distribution depend on:

- **Blood flow** – Highly perfused organs (heart, liver, kidneys) receive drugs faster than fatty tissues or skin.
- **Solubility** – Fat-soluble drugs easily cross membranes, while water-soluble drugs may need transport mechanisms.

- **Protein Binding** – Some drugs bind to proteins in the blood (like albumin). Only the free drug is active; the bound drug is inactive until released.

Metabolism: How the Body Processes Drugs

Metabolism (or biotransformation) refers to how the body chemically alters drugs to prepare them for elimination.

How Drugs Are Metabolized

Most drugs are broken down by liver enzymes into inactive forms that can be excreted.

Some drugs are converted into active metabolites, meaning they become more potent after metabolism.

Prodrugs are inactive when taken but become active only after metabolism.

Factors Affecting Metabolism

- **Liver Health** – Liver diseases (like cirrhosis) slow metabolism, causing drugs to stay in the system longer.
- **Genetics** – Some people metabolize drugs faster or slower due to genetic variations.
- **Environment** – Smoking, stress, and diet can speed up or slow down metabolism.
- **Age** – Infants have immature livers and metabolize drugs slowly, while elderly patients experience slower metabolism due to reduced liver function.

Excretion: Removing Drugs from the Body

Once metabolized, drugs need to be eliminated. The kidneys are the primary organ responsible for drug excretion through urine, but other pathways include:

- **Lungs** – Some drugs (like anesthetic gases) are exhaled.

- **Sweat & Saliva** – Small amounts of drugs exit through sweat or saliva.
- **Breast Milk** – Some medications pass into breast milk, affecting nursing infants.
- **Feces** – Certain drugs are eliminated through bile and passed in the stool.

Half-Life & Drug Duration

A drug's half-life is the time it takes for half of the drug to be eliminated from the body. This helps determine:

- How often a drug should be taken (short half-life = frequent doses; long half-life = fewer doses).
- How long a drug stays active in the body.

Steady State & Drug Dosing

- If a drug is taken at regular intervals, it reaches a steady level in the blood after 4–5 half-lives.
- Example: A drug with a 6-hour half-life reaches steady state after 24–30 hours of regular dosing.

Onset, Peak, and Duration of Drug Effects

- **Onset of Action** – Time from administration to when the drug starts working.
- **Peak Concentration** – The highest level of the drug in the bloodstream.
- **Duration of Action** – How long the drug remains effective.

Each drug has a unique onset, peak, and duration, which influences how and when it should be taken.

1.3. Pharmacodynamics: How Drugs Work in the Body

Pharmacodynamics is the science of how drugs interact with the body to produce their effects. Essentially, it explains what a drug does once it reaches its target—whether it stimulates, blocks, or modifies a biological response.

At the cellular level, drugs interact with proteins, enzymes, and receptors found on cell membranes or inside cells. This interaction is what triggers the therapeutic (or sometimes adverse) effects of a drug.

How Drugs Influence Cell Function

Drugs can't create new functions in the body—they can only modify existing ones. They do this in two primary ways:

- Changing the physical or chemical environment of the cell.
- Interacting with receptors (specialized sites on cell membranes or inside cells).

Activating a Response: Agonists

Some drugs activate receptors to produce an effect—these are called agonists.

- Agonists have an affinity (strong attraction) for a receptor.
- Once bound, they stimulate a biological response.
- The intensity of the effect depends on the drug's ability to activate the receptor—this is called its intrinsic activity.

Example: Morphine is an agonist that binds to opioid receptors to relieve pain.

Blocking a Response: Antagonists

Other drugs bind to receptors but don't activate them—these are called antagonists. Instead, they block or reduce the action of natural substances or other drugs.

- **Competitive antagonists** – These compete with agonists for the same receptor. If more of an agonist is given, it can overcome the antagonist's effects.
- **Noncompetitive antagonists** – These permanently block the receptor, making it impossible for an agonist to bind, regardless of the dose.

Example: Beta-blockers prevent adrenaline from binding to heart receptors, reducing heart rate and blood pressure.

Selective vs. Nonselective Drugs

- Selective drugs target specific receptors, causing fewer side effects.
- Nonselective drugs affect multiple receptors, leading to broader effects (both beneficial and harmful).

Example:

- Selective beta-blockers (like atenolol) target only the heart.
- Nonselective beta-blockers (like propranolol) affect both the heart and lungs, which can cause respiratory issues in asthma patients.

Understanding Drug Potency and Safety

Drug Potency

Potency refers to how much of a drug is needed to achieve a specific effect.

- If Drug X produces the same effect as Drug Y at a lower dose, then Drug X is more potent.

- A highly potent drug requires smaller doses to be effective.

Therapeutic Index: Measuring Drug Safety

Every drug has a therapeutic index, which measures the gap between an effective dose and a toxic dose.

- Narrow therapeutic index – A small difference between an effective and toxic dose (higher risk of overdose).
- Wide therapeutic index – A larger safety margin (lower risk of overdose).

Example:

- Warfarin (blood thinner) has a narrow therapeutic index, meaning it requires careful monitoring.
- Ibuprofen has a wide therapeutic index, meaning over-the-counter use is generally safe.

1.4. Pharmacotherapeutics: How Drugs Are Used to Treat Diseases

Pharmacotherapeutics focuses on using drugs to prevent, treat, or manage medical conditions. When choosing a medication, healthcare providers consider:

- How effective the drug is for the condition.
- The patient's overall health and medical history.
- Possible drug interactions or side effects.

Types of Drug Therapy

The type of therapy depends on the patient's condition and treatment goals.

1. **Acute Therapy** – Used for severe, life-threatening conditions that require immediate intervention (e.g., IV antibiotics for sepsis).

2. **Empiric Therapy** – Based on past experience rather than lab tests (e.g., prescribing antibiotics for suspected bacterial infections).
3. **Maintenance Therapy** – Helps manage chronic conditions without curing them (e.g., insulin for diabetes, blood pressure meds for hypertension).
4. **Supplemental Therapy** – Replaces missing substances in the body (e.g., iron supplements for anemia, hormone therapy for thyroid disorders).
5. **Supportive Therapy** – Helps maintain vital functions while the body recovers (e.g., IV fluids for dehydration).
6. **Palliative Therapy** – Focuses on comfort rather than curing the disease (e.g., pain management in terminal cancer patients).

Personalized Drug Responses

Every patient reacts to medication differently based on factors like:

- **Genetics** – Some people metabolize drugs faster or slower than others.
- **Age** – Children and elderly patients often need adjusted doses.
- **Lifestyle factors** – Diet, alcohol, and smoking can alter drug effectiveness.

Drug Tolerance and Dependence

Drug Tolerance: When Medications Become Less Effective

Over time, some drugs become less effective, requiring higher doses to achieve the same result.

- Example: Opioid users may develop tolerance and need higher doses for pain relief.

Drug Dependence: When the Body Relies on a Drug

- **Physical dependence** – The body experiences withdrawal symptoms when the drug is stopped.
- **Psychological dependence** – The patient feels the need to keep taking the drug to relieve stress or discomfort.

1.5. Drug Interactions: When Medications Affect Each Other

Taking multiple medications can change how they work, sometimes leading to dangerous effects.

Types of Drug Interactions

1. **Additive Effect** – When two drugs with similar effects are taken together, their effects combine.
   Example: Taking two pain relievers (Tylenol + Advil) can provide better pain relief with lower doses.
2. **Synergistic Effect (Potentiation)** – When one drug enhances the effect of another.
   Example: Alcohol increases the sedative effects of sleeping pills, making them more potent than expected.
3. **Antagonistic Effect** – When one drug blocks or reduces the effect of another.
   Example: Some antacids reduce the absorption of antibiotics, making them less effective.

How Food and Drugs Interact

Food Can Affect Drug Absorption

- High-fat meals slow down drug absorption.
- Some medications need food to prevent stomach irritation (e.g., ibuprofen).
- Others should be taken on an empty stomach for better absorption (e.g., thyroid medications).

Dangerous Food-Drug Interactions

- Tyramine-containing foods (cheese, wine) can cause dangerous blood pressure spikes when combined with certain antidepressants (MAO inhibitors).
- Grapefruit juice can increase drug levels in the blood, leading to toxic effects (e.g., some statins, blood pressure medications).

How Drugs Affect Lab Tests

Certain medications can alter test results, leading to false readings.

- Diuretics may lower potassium levels.
- Antibiotics can interfere with blood cultures.
- Steroids can raise blood sugar levels, mimicking diabetes.

1.6. Adverse Drug Reactions: When Medications Cause Harm

Every drug is designed to produce a specific therapeutic effect—its intended benefit. However, not all drug responses are positive. Adverse drug reactions (ADRs) occur when a medication triggers unwanted, harmful effects in the body. These reactions can range from mild and temporary (such as nausea or drowsiness) to severe and life-threatening (such as organ failure or anaphylaxis). Some ADRs appear immediately after taking a drug, while others develop over time with continued use.

What Causes Adverse Drug Reactions?

ADRs generally fall into two categories:

1. Dose-Related Reactions

These reactions occur when the dose of a drug is too high for the body to handle, leading to exaggerated effects. They are often predictable and can be managed by adjusting the dose.

Common dose-related reactions include:

- **Secondary effects** – A drug achieves its primary goal but also causes unintended side effects.
  Example: Morphine relieves pain but also causes constipation and drowsiness.
- **Hypersusceptibility** – Some people are more sensitive to a drug than others, leading to an intense response even at normal doses.
  Example: A small dose of a sedative may cause excessive drowsiness in an elderly patient.
- **Overdose** – Taking too much of a drug (either accidentally or intentionally) can lead to toxicity.
  Example: A high dose of acetaminophen can cause liver damage.
- **Iatrogenic effects** – Some drugs mimic disease symptoms, making it seem like a patient has a new illness.
  Example: Long-term corticosteroid use can cause osteoporosis.

2. Patient Sensitivity-Related Reactions

Some adverse reactions occur because an individual's body reacts unusually to a drug, even at normal doses. These reactions are less predictable and vary from person to person.

Two major types of patient-specific ADRs include:

- Allergic Reactions – When the immune system mistakes a drug for a harmful substance, leading to an allergic response.
  Mild symptoms: Rash, itching, hives.
  Severe symptoms: Anaphylaxis, a life-threatening reaction that can cause breathing difficulties, swelling of the throat, and a sudden drop in blood pressure.
- Idiosyncratic Responses – Rare and unpredictable reactions that aren't related to a drug's normal function. These often have a genetic basis.
  Example: A drug meant to lower blood pressure unexpectedly causes severe muscle cramps in one patient but not others.

1.7. The Nursing Process: Ensuring Safe and Effective Drug Administration

One of the most critical aspects of modern nursing is following a structured nursing process to ensure safe medication use. This process is a problem-solving approach that helps nurses provide the best possible care while minimizing medication errors and adverse effects.

The five key steps of the nursing process are:

4. Assessment – Gathering patient information.
5. Nursing Diagnosis – Identifying health concerns.
6. Planning – Setting treatment goals.
7. Implementation – Administering medications and treatments.
8. Evaluation – Monitoring the patient's response.

Step 1: Assessment – Gathering Patient Information

Before giving any medication, nurses must assess the patient's health status to ensure the drug is safe and appropriate.

Key assessment factors include:

- **Medical history** – Past and current illnesses, allergies, and previous adverse drug reactions.
- **Current medications** – Prescription drugs, over-the-counter medications, supplements, and herbal products.
- **Lab tests and vital signs** – Some drugs require monitoring of kidney function, liver enzymes, blood pressure, or heart rate before administration.

Step 2: Nursing Diagnosis – Identifying Potential Problems

A nursing diagnosis is a clinical judgment about the patient's health condition that guides treatment decisions.

For example:

- A patient taking a blood thinner may have a diagnosis of "Risk for bleeding".
- A patient on opioid pain medication may have a diagnosis of "Risk for respiratory depression".

Nurses use these diagnoses to anticipate and prevent complications before they occur.

Step 3: Planning – Setting Goals for Treatment

A care plan is developed to ensure that drug therapy meets the patient's needs safely and effectively. It includes:

- **Expected outcomes** – What is the goal of the drug therapy? (e.g., "Patient's pain level will decrease from 8/10 to 3/10 within 30 minutes of receiving morphine.")
- **Nursing interventions** – What steps should be taken to achieve the goal? (e.g., "Monitor respiratory rate and level of sedation after morphine administration.")

Step 4: Implementation – Administering Medications and Providing Care

This is when nurses put the care plan into action. The implementation phase includes:

Administering medications correctly – Following the "Five Rights of Medication Administration":

1. Right Patient – Verify the patient's identity.
2. Right Drug – Ensure the correct medication is given.
3. Right Dose – Give the exact prescribed amount.
4. Right Time – Administer the drug at the correct time.
5. Right Route – Ensure the drug is given the right way (oral, IV, etc.).

Patient education – Teaching the patient about possible side effects, food interactions, and what to do if they miss a dose.

Monitoring for side effects – Watching for any signs of adverse drug reactions.

Step 5: Evaluation – Monitoring the Patient's Response

After giving a medication, nurses must evaluate its effectiveness and watch for side effects or complications.

- Did the drug work as expected?
- Are there any adverse effects?
- Does the patient need a dosage adjustment or a different medication?

If the patient isn't responding well to the drug, the nurse communicates with the healthcare provider to adjust treatment as needed.

Chapter 2: Drugs for Autonomic Nervous System

2.1. Drugs and the Autonomic Nervous System: How Medications Affect Body Functions

The autonomic nervous system (ANS) controls the body's involuntary functions, such as heart rate, breathing, digestion, and blood pressure. It works through two main divisions:

- The Sympathetic Nervous System (fight-or-flight) – Prepares the body for action.
- The Parasympathetic Nervous System (rest-and-digest) – Helps the body relax and recover.

When these systems become overactive or underactive, medications are used to restore balance. The main types of drugs affecting the ANS include:

- **Cholinergic drugs** – Stimulate the parasympathetic system.
- **Anticholinergic drugs** – Block parasympathetic activity.
- **Adrenergic drugs** – Activate the sympathetic system.
- **Adrenergic blocking drugs** – Reduce sympathetic activity.

These drugs help regulate heart function, digestion, respiratory health, and more.

2.2. Cholinergic Drugs: Activating the Parasympathetic System

Cholinergic drugs enhance the effects of acetylcholine, the neurotransmitter responsible for stimulating the parasympathetic nervous system. These drugs are also called parasympathomimetics because they mimic the natural effects of parasympathetic nerve activity.

How Cholinergic Drugs Work

There are two main types of cholinergic drugs:

1. **Cholinergic Agonists** – Directly stimulate receptors to act like acetylcholine.
2. **Anticholinesterase Drugs** – Prevent acetylcholine from breaking down, allowing it to work longer.

Common cholinergic agonists include:

- **Acetylcholine** (not to be confused with the natural neurotransmitter).
- **Bethanechol** – Used to treat urinary retention.
- **Carbachol & Pilocarpine** – Help reduce eye pressure in glaucoma patients.

How Cholinergic Drugs Move Through the Body (Pharmacokinetics)

The way these drugs enter and travel through the body depends on their formulation and how they're administered:

- Common methods: Eye drops, oral tablets, and subcutaneous (under the skin) injections.
- Why not IV or IM? These drugs are broken down too quickly in the bloodstream and can cause a cholinergic crisis (dangerous muscle weakness and breathing difficulties).
- How fast do they work? They start working within 2 hours, and food can slow down their absorption.
- How are they removed? They're broken down by cholinesterase and excreted by the kidneys.

What Cholinergic Drugs Do in the Body (Pharmacodynamics)

By acting like acetylcholine, cholinergic drugs cause the following effects:

- Increased saliva production.
- Slower heart rate (bradycardia).
- Lower blood pressure (vasodilation).
- Narrowed airways (bronchoconstriction).
- Increased digestion and bladder activity.
- Smaller pupils (miosis), which reduces eye pressure.

Why Are Cholinergic Drugs Used? (Pharmacotherapeutics)

Cholinergic drugs help manage conditions such as:

- Weak bladder conditions & urinary retention (Bethanechol).
- Digestive issues like post-surgery bowel inactivity.
- Glaucoma – Helps reduce eye pressure.
- Dry mouth from radiation therapy or autoimmune disorders (Sjögren's syndrome).

Drug Interactions: What to Watch Out For

Cholinergic drugs can interact with other medications, either increasing or reducing their effects:

- Other cholinergic drugs (like anticholinesterase medications) increase toxicity risk.
- Anticholinergic drugs (such as atropine) reduce the effects of cholinergic drugs.
- Quinidine (a heart medication) makes cholinergic drugs less effective.

Possible Side Effects & Risks

Because cholinergic drugs activate the parasympathetic system, they can cause side effects throughout the body:

- **Digestive issues** – Nausea, vomiting, diarrhea, cramps.
- **Heart and blood pressure changes** – Slow heart rate, low blood pressure.
- **Breathing difficulties** – Narrowed airways, shortness of breath.
- **Frequent urination** – Due to increased bladder activity.
- **Excess saliva and sweating** – Overstimulation of glands.

Nursing Process: Safe Administration of Cholinergic Drugs

To ensure safe and effective use, nurses follow a structured care process:

1. Assessment

- Check if the patient has urinary retention, digestive issues, or glaucoma.
- Monitor for pre-existing conditions (e.g., asthma, heart problems) that could worsen with cholinergic drugs.

2. Nursing Diagnosis

- Risk for respiratory issues (due to increased secretions).
- Impaired urinary elimination (if the drug works too well and leads to excessive urination).

3. Planning Goals

- Ensure safe oxygen levels.
- Restore normal urination and digestion.
- Monitor therapeutic effects and side effects.

4. Implementation (Giving the Medication)

- Follow dosing instructions (some must be taken before meals).

- Monitor for side effects and report any breathing difficulties.

- Does the patient's condition improve?
- Are there any adverse effects that need attention?
- Can the patient or caregiver administer the medication correctly?

Anticholinesterase Drugs: Enhancing Acetylcholine Activity

These drugs work by blocking the enzyme acetylcholinesterase, which normally breaks down acetylcholine. This allows acetylcholine to stay active longer, enhancing its effects.

Types of Anticholinesterase Drugs

There are two major types:

1. Reversible – Short-term effects, used in medical treatment. Examples: Donepezil, Neostigmine, Pyridostigmine, Rivastigmine.
2. Irreversible – Long-lasting effects, mostly found in pesticides and chemical warfare agents.

How These Drugs Work in the Body

- **Absorption:** Quickly absorbed from the GI tract, skin, and mucous membranes.
- **Metabolism & Excretion:** Broken down by enzymes in the liver and plasma, then excreted in urine.
- **How Long Do They Last?** Some work for hours (like neostigmine), while others can last for days or weeks.

What Are Anticholinesterase Drugs Used For?

These drugs treat conditions where acetylcholine activity is too low, such as:

- **Glaucoma** – Lowers eye pressure.

- **Weak bladder and intestines** – Helps improve muscle tone.
- **Myasthenia gravis** – Boosts muscle contraction.
- **Alzheimer's disease** – Slows cognitive decline (Donepezil, Rivastigmine).
- **Reversing toxic overdoses** – Used as antidotes for certain poisons.

Drug Interactions: What to Avoid

- Mixing with other cholinergic drugs can increase toxicity.
- Anticholinergic drugs (like atropine) can reduce effectiveness.
- Certain seizure medications and steroids can change how the drug is broken down.

Possible Side Effects

Most side effects happen because acetylcholine activity is too high, leading to:

- **Heart issues** – Irregular heartbeat, low blood pressure.
- **Digestive problems** – Nausea, vomiting, diarrhea.
- **Neurological effects** – Seizures, headaches, insomnia.
- **Breathing issues** – Wheezing, chest tightness.

Nursing Considerations for Anticholinesterase Drugs

1. Monitor for conditions that may worsen, such as blockages in the intestines or urinary tract.
2. Assess breathing and heart function before giving the drug.
3. Ensure the patient understands how to take the medication correctly.

Fluid Balance and Nursing Considerations

Managing fluids in the body is critical when administering medications that affect the autonomic nervous system. Proper assessment and intervention help ensure safe and effective treatment.

Assessment: Checking Fluid and Organ Function

- **Monitor urinary retention and bladder distention** – Check how much fluid the patient is drinking and when they last urinated.
- **Assess for potential digestive issues (paralytic ileus)** – Listen for bowel sounds, check for bloating, and assess stool patterns.

Key Nursing Diagnoses

- Impaired gas exchange – If the patient has difficulty breathing due to bronchospasms or respiratory paralysis.
- Impaired tissue integrity – Some medications, like anticholinergic drugs, may cause skin breakdown or poor circulation.
- Impaired urinary elimination – Certain drugs may affect bladder control, leading to urinary retention or increased frequency.

Planning Goals: What We Want to Achieve

1. Ensure the patient maintains proper oxygen levels.
2. Restore normal urinary and bowel function.
3. Observe positive effects of anticholinesterase drugs.
4. Educate the patient on correct medication use.

Implementation: Actions for Safe Medication Use

- Give anticholinesterase drugs before meals, unless directed otherwise.
- Monitor for side effects and report any unusual reactions.
- Be extra cautious with elderly patients, as they are more sensitive to these drugs.
- Encourage deep breathing and positioning techniques to promote better lung function.
- Check for urinary retention and support patients in following a medication schedule.

- Educate patients and caregivers on proper medication use and possible side effects.

Evaluation: Measuring Patient Progress

- The patient's condition improves with treatment.
- The patient maintains normal breathing without distress.
- The patient urinates and defecates normally.
- The patient and caregivers understand how to use medications correctly.

2.3. Anticholinergic Drugs: Blocking the Parasympathetic Nervous System

Anticholinergic drugs, also known as cholinergic blockers, inhibit the effects of acetylcholine on the parasympathetic nervous system. This results in:

- Increased heart rate.
- Reduced digestive secretions.
- Relaxed bladder muscles.
- Dilated pupils.

They are widely used to treat respiratory issues, heart problems, digestive disorders, and more.

How They Work: Targeting Muscarinic Receptors

- These drugs don't block all cholinergic receptors—only the muscarinic receptors.
- Muscarinic receptors control involuntary muscle movements and secretions, meaning these drugs reduce excessive secretions, slow digestion, and speed up heart rate.

Common Anticholinergic Medications

Belladonna Alkaloids (Natural Sources):

- Atropine – Used for heart rhythm problems and pre-surgery.
- Scopolamine – Helps with motion sickness and nausea.

- Ipratropium – Treats respiratory conditions like asthma and COPD.

Synthetic Versions:

- Glycopyrrolate – Reduces saliva and stomach acid production.
- Methscopolamine – Used for digestive issues.

Tertiary Amines (Newer Anticholinergics with Fewer Side Effects):

- Benztropine – Used for Parkinson's disease.
- Oxybutynin & Tolterodine – Treat overactive bladder.
- Trihexyphenidyl – Used for movement disorders.

How These Drugs Move Through the Body (Pharmacokinetics)

- Well-absorbed through the eyes, stomach, mucous membranes, and skin.
- Fast-acting when given IV (Atropine starts working immediately).
- Metabolized in the liver and excreted mostly by the kidneys.
- Tertiary amines (like benztropine) are more selective and have fewer side effects than older drugs.

How Anticholinergic Drugs Affect the Body (Pharmacodynamics)

- The effects depend on dose, condition, and organ targeted.
- In the brain, low doses can be stimulating, while high doses can be sedating.
- In conditions like Parkinson's disease, these drugs help reduce excessive movement and tremors.

Common Uses of Anticholinergic Drugs (Pharmacotherapeutics)

- **GI issues** – Used to relax stomach and bladder muscles, helping treat:
  Irritable bowel syndrome (IBS).
  Overactive bladder (Oxybutynin).
- **Pre-Surgery** – Atropine is given before surgery to:
  Reduce saliva and mucus production.
  Prevent slow heart rate during anesthesia.
- **Motion Sickness** – Scopolamine helps prevent nausea and dizziness.
- **Heart Conditions** – Atropine raises heart rate in bradycardia (slow heart rate).
- **Eye Exams** – Used to dilate pupils for vision tests and surgeries.

Drug Interactions: What to Watch For

Some medications increase or reduce the effects of anticholinergic drugs:

Medications That Increase Effects (Higher Risk of Side Effects)

- Antidepressants (Amitriptyline, Nortriptyline).
- Antipsychotics (Haloperidol, Clozapine).
- Muscle relaxants (Cyclobenzaprine).

Medications That Decrease Effects (Lower Drug Effectiveness)

- Cholinergic drugs (Bethanechol, Neostigmine) – Counteract anticholinergic effects.

Potential Side Effects & Risks

Anticholinergic drugs come with several side effects, which can vary based on dosage:

- Dry mouth – Due to reduced saliva production.
- Blurred vision – From pupil dilation.

- Increased heart rate (tachycardia).
- Constipation & urinary retention – Caused by reduced digestive and bladder activity.
- Confusion & memory issues – More common in elderly patients.

High doses can cause serious reactions, including hallucinations, extreme confusion, and high fever.

Nursing Process: Ensuring Safe Anticholinergic Drug Use

1. Assessment

- Check for heart, bladder, or digestive conditions before giving these drugs.
- Identify conditions where these drugs should be avoided (e.g., glaucoma, enlarged prostate, or myasthenia gravis).

2. Key Nursing Diagnoses

- **Risk for urinary retention** – Due to drug effects on the bladder.
- **Risk for constipation** – Due to slowed digestion.
- **Potential confusion or memory issues** – Especially in elderly patients.

3. Planning Goals

- Ensure symptom relief without causing severe side effects.
- Maintain normal heart rate and breathing patterns.
- Prevent serious complications like dehydration from reduced saliva production.

4. Implementation: Administering the Medication Safely

- Follow the correct dosage schedule (some drugs must be taken with food).
- Monitor heart rate, urine output, and vision changes.

- Watch for signs of overdose (delirium, fever, extreme dry mouth).
- Help manage dry mouth with lozenges and increased fluid intake.

5. Evaluation: Measuring Patient Progress

- Does the patient's condition improve?
- Are side effects manageable?
- Can the patient safely use the medication at home?

2.4. Adrenergic Drugs: Activating the Sympathetic Nervous System

Adrenergic drugs, also known as sympathomimetics, mimic the fight-or-flight response by stimulating the sympathetic nervous system (SNS). These drugs help regulate heart rate, blood pressure, breathing, and energy levels, making them useful in treating conditions like asthma, low blood pressure, and cardiac arrest.

How Adrenergic Drugs Are Classified

There are two main ways to classify adrenergic drugs:

1. By Chemical Structure

- **Catecholamines** – These include natural (produced by the body) and synthetic forms that directly stimulate the nervous system.
- **Noncatecholamines** – These are longer-lasting and can be used for bronchodilation, decongestion, and blood pressure control.

2. By Mode of Action

- **Direct-acting** – Work directly on the target organ (e.g., epinephrine).
- **Indirect-acting** – Trigger the release of natural neurotransmitters (e.g., amphetamines).

- **Dual-acting** – Have both direct and indirect effects (e.g., ephedrine).

Catecholamines: Powerful, Fast-Acting Sympathomimetics

Catecholamines are potent adrenergic drugs that cause:

- Increased heart rate.
- Constricted blood vessels (raising blood pressure).
- Dilated airways (improving breathing).

Common Catecholamines

- Dobutamine – Used to improve heart function.
- Dopamine – Helps increase blood flow to the kidneys and improves heart function.
- Epinephrine (Adrenaline) – Used in cardiac arrest, anaphylaxis, and severe asthma attacks.
- Norepinephrine – Used to raise dangerously low blood pressure.
- Isoproterenol – A synthetic drug that stimulates the heart and lungs.

How Catecholamines Work in the Body (Pharmacokinetics)

Absorption & Administration

- Cannot be taken orally – Digestive enzymes break them down too quickly.
- Given sublingually (under the tongue) for rapid absorption.
- Injected intramuscularly (IM) or intravenously (IV) for emergency situations.

Distribution & Metabolism

- Widely distributed throughout the body.

- Metabolized mainly in the liver, kidneys, lungs, and gastrointestinal (GI) tract.

Excretion

- Mostly eliminated through urine.
- Small amounts may be found in breast milk or feces.

How Catecholamines Affect the Body (Pharmacodynamics)

Impact on Organs

- Heart – Strengthens heart contractions (positive inotropic effect) and increases heart rate (positive chronotropic effect).
- Lungs – Opens up airways (bronchodilation) to make breathing easier.
- Blood Vessels – Constricts blood vessels (vasoconstriction) to raise blood pressure.

Effect on Heart Rhythms

- Increased electrical activity – Can improve cardiac function but may also lead to irregular heartbeats (arrhythmias).
- Epinephrine may cause the heart's Purkinje fibers to fire randomly, leading to dangerous heart rhythms.

Medical Uses of Adrenergic Drugs (Pharmacotherapeutics)

Heart & Blood Pressure Regulation

- Low Blood Pressure (Hypotension) – Norepinephrine is used to raise blood pressure in critically ill patients.
- Bradycardia (Slow Heart Rate) – Dopamine and epinephrine help increase heart rate.
- Cardiac Arrest – Epinephrine is used in advanced cardiac life support (ACLS) protocols.

Respiratory Conditions

- Asthma & COPD – Beta-2 adrenergic drugs (like albuterol) help open airways.
- Severe Allergic Reactions (Anaphylaxis) – Epinephrine reverses airway swelling and low blood pressure.

Kidney Function & Blood Flow

- Dopamine at low doses improves kidney blood flow, helping prevent kidney failure in critically ill patients.

Drug Interactions: What to Watch For

Certain drugs can enhance or reduce the effects of catecholamines:

Medications That Increase Effects (Risk of Overstimulation)

- Alpha-blockers (like phentolamine) – Can cause a dangerous drop in blood pressure.
- Tricyclic Antidepressants – May lead to severe high blood pressure.
- Other Adrenergic Drugs – May increase heart rate and blood pressure too much.

Medications That Decrease Effects

- Beta-blockers (like propranolol) – Can block the effects of catecholamines and cause bronchoconstriction in asthma patients.

Potential Side Effects of Catecholamines

While adrenergic drugs save lives in emergencies, they can also cause serious side effects:

- Restlessness & anxiety.
- Headaches & dizziness.
- Palpitations & irregular heart rhythms.

- High blood pressure (hypertension) – May lead to stroke in extreme cases.
- Tissue damage if an IV injection leaks into surrounding tissues.

High doses or prolonged use may lead to severe complications, including stroke or heart failure.

Nursing Process: Ensuring Safe Use of Adrenergic Drugs

1. Assessment: Checking the Patient's Condition

- Monitor blood pressure, heart rate, oxygen levels, and kidney function before starting treatment.
- Use continuous ECG monitoring for IV-administered catecholamines.

2. Nursing Diagnoses

- Risk for high blood pressure or irregular heart rhythms.
- Risk for tissue damage if the drug leaks from an IV.
- Deficient knowledge of drug use – Educate the patient and caregivers.

3. Planning Goals

- Maintain stable blood pressure and heart rate.
- Ensure proper blood circulation to vital organs.
- Prevent complications from drug interactions or overdose.

4. Implementation: Administering Adrenergic Drugs Safely

- Correct dehydration first – If a patient is low on fluids, the drug may not work as expected.
- Use a central venous catheter for IV administration – Reduces the risk of tissue damage.
- Monitor for early signs of overdose, such as severe anxiety, chest pain, or confusion.

- Does the patient's condition improve?
- Are there any dangerous side effects?
- Does the patient understand how and when to use the medication?

Noncatecholamine Adrenergic Drugs: Longer-Lasting Options

Unlike catecholamines, noncatecholamines:

- Last longer in the body.
- Can be taken orally.
- Have different effects, such as bronchodilation, decongestion, and smooth muscle relaxation.

Examples & Uses

- Phenylephrine – Used to constrict blood vessels and reduce swelling.
- Albuterol & Salmeterol – Open airways in asthma and COPD patients.
- Terbutaline – Relaxes muscles to prevent preterm labor.

Warning: Some noncatecholamines may cause dangerously high blood pressure if taken with antidepressants or MAO inhibitors.

2.5. Adrenergic Blocking Drugs: Slowing Down the Sympathetic Response

Adrenergic blocking drugs, also known as sympatholytics, work opposite to adrenergic (sympathomimetic) drugs. Instead of stimulating the fight-or-flight response, these drugs block or slow down sympathetic nervous system activity.

They achieve this by:

- Interrupting the action of adrenergic drugs.

- Reducing the amount of norepinephrine available in the body.
- Preventing adrenergic stimulation at receptor sites.

These drugs are commonly used to treat high blood pressure, heart disease, and circulation problems.

Types of Adrenergic Blocking Drugs

Adrenergic blockers are classified based on the receptors they target:

- Alpha-adrenergic blockers (Alpha Blockers) – Affect blood vessels.
- Beta-adrenergic blockers (Beta Blockers) – Affect the heart and lungs.

Alpha-Adrenergic Blockers: Relaxing Blood Vessels

How They Work

Alpha blockers block the effects of epinephrine and norepinephrine at alpha-receptor sites, leading to:

- Relaxation of blood vessel walls.
- Improved blood flow and circulation.
- Lower blood pressure.

Common Alpha Blockers

- Prazosin & Doxazosin – Used for high blood pressure and benign prostatic hyperplasia (BPH).
- Terazosin – Helps with urine flow in men with prostate enlargement.
- Phentolamine – Used in emergency situations for severe high blood pressure.

How They Move Through the Body (Pharmacokinetics)

- Absorbed erratically when taken orally.
- Faster absorption when taken sublingually (under the tongue).

- Varied onset and duration, depending on the drug.

What Alpha Blockers Do in the Body (Pharmacodynamics)

Alpha blockers work by blocking norepinephrine's ability to tighten blood vessels, which leads to vasodilation (wider blood vessels), allowing for better circulation and lower blood pressure.

However, the effect depends on the patient's position:

- Lying down → Minimal blood pressure drop.
- Standing up quickly → Blood may pool in the legs, causing dizziness or fainting (orthostatic hypotension).

Why Alpha Blockers Are Used (Pharmacotherapeutics)

Common Conditions Treated

- Hypertension (High Blood Pressure) – Helps lower blood pressure by relaxing blood vessels.
- Circulation Disorders – Used for conditions like Raynaud's disease and frostbite, which cause poor blood flow to the hands and feet.
- Pheochromocytoma – A rare adrenal tumor that releases too much adrenaline, causing dangerously high blood pressure.
- Migraines & Vascular Headaches – Alpha blockers can relieve migraine symptoms by improving blood flow.
- Benign Prostatic Hyperplasia (BPH) – Helps relax the muscles around the prostate, making urination easier for men with an enlarged prostate.

Drug Interactions: What to Watch For

Alpha blockers can interact with other medications, leading to exaggerated effects:

- Taking prazosin with diuretics or beta-blockers → Increases the risk of fainting.

- Mixing terazosin with antihypertensive drugs → May cause dangerously low blood pressure.
- Caffeine & Macrolide Antibiotics (when taken with ergotamine, a migraine treatment) → Increases drug effects, leading to excessive dilation of blood vessels.

Risk Alert: Taking nitroglycerin with alpha blockers may cause severe low blood pressure and dizziness.

Side Effects of Alpha Blockers

Most side effects come from blood vessels expanding too much:

- Orthostatic Hypotension (dizziness when standing up).
- Slow or fast heart rate (bradycardia/tachycardia).
- Swelling (edema).
- Shortness of breath.
- Flushed skin and light-headedness.
- Chest pain (angina).

In rare cases, excessive blood vessel dilation can lead to heart attack or stroke.

Nursing Process: Ensuring Safe Use of Alpha Blockers

1. Assessment: Checking the Patient's Condition

- Monitor blood pressure and heart rate regularly.
- Watch for signs of dizziness, fainting, or swelling.
- Assess the patient's understanding of the medication and any concerns.

2. Nursing Diagnoses

- Risk for falls related to low blood pressure.
- Risk for fluid retention and swelling.
- Deficient knowledge of medication use.

3. Planning Goals

- Ensure stable blood pressure and good circulation.

- Minimize dizziness and risk of fainting.
- Help patients understand how and when to take their medication.

4. Implementation: Giving the Medication Safely

- Give medication at bedtime to reduce the risk of fainting.
- Start with a low dose and increase gradually.
- Encourage slow movements (especially when standing up).
- For migraines, give ergotamine at the first sign of symptoms.

5. Evaluation: Measuring Treatment Success

- Has the patient's blood pressure improved?
- Are side effects minimal and manageable?
- Does the patient understand how to take the medication safely?

Beta Blockers: Slowing the Heart and Reducing Stress on the Body

Beta-adrenergic blockers, commonly known as beta blockers, prevent the effects of adrenaline by blocking beta-receptor sites.

These drugs:

- Lower heart rate and blood pressure.
- Reduce oxygen demand on the heart.
- Help treat heart disease, anxiety, and migraines.

Types of Beta Blockers

- Nonselective beta blockers – Affect both beta-1 (heart) and beta-2 (lungs) receptors (e.g., propranolol, carvedilol).
- Selective beta blockers – Primarily affect beta-1 receptors in the heart, making them safer for people with lung diseases (e.g., metoprolol, atenolol).

Common Uses of Beta Blockers

- High Blood Pressure & Heart Disease – Lower blood pressure and protect the heart.
- Anxiety & Tremors – Used for stage fright and essential tremors.
- Migraine Prevention – Helps reduce frequency and severity of migraines.
- Glaucoma – Lowers eye pressure.

Drug Interactions: What to Avoid with Beta Blockers

Warning: Certain drugs can make beta blockers more dangerous:

- Calcium channel blockers & digoxin – May cause severe low heart rate.
- Asthma medications (like theophylline) – Can lose effectiveness when combined with beta blockers.
- Diabetes medications – Beta blockers can hide symptoms of low blood sugar, making it harder to detect hypoglycemia.

Potential Side Effects of Beta Blockers

- Fatigue & dizziness.
- Slow heart rate (bradycardia).
- Shortness of breath (especially in people with asthma or COPD).
- Cold hands and feet due to reduced circulation.
- Depression or mood changes.

Beta blockers should never be stopped suddenly—doing so can cause a rebound effect, leading to high blood pressure or heart attack.

Chapter 3: Neurologic and Neuromuscular Drugs

3.1. Medications for the Nervous and Neuromuscular Systems

The nervous system and neuromuscular system play a vital role in movement, sensation, and overall body function. When these systems are affected by disease or injury, medications are often needed to manage symptoms and improve quality of life.

This chapter covers different types of neurologic and neuromuscular drugs, including:

- Skeletal muscle relaxants – Help relieve muscle spasms and stiffness.
- Neuromuscular blocking agents – Used during surgery to prevent involuntary movements.
- Antiparkinsonian drugs – Help manage Parkinson's disease symptoms.
- Anticonvulsants – Prevent seizures in people with epilepsy.
- Antimigraine drugs – Reduce the frequency and severity of migraines.

The nervous system consists of:

- The Central Nervous System (CNS) – Includes the brain and spinal cord.
- The Peripheral Nervous System (PNS) – Includes somatic (voluntary) and autonomic (involuntary) functions.

The neuromuscular system connects nerves to muscles, allowing movement and reflex responses. When neurologic or muscular disorders occur, medications can help relax muscles, control nerve signals, or improve movement.

3.2. Skeletal Muscle Relaxants: Relieving Muscle Tension and Spasms

What Are Skeletal Muscle Relaxants?

These medications help reduce muscle pain, stiffness, and spasms caused by:

- Muscle injuries or inflammation.
- Neurologic disorders (like multiple sclerosis, cerebral palsy, or stroke).
- Spinal cord injuries that lead to paralysis or severe spasticity.

There are two main types of muscle relaxants:

1. Centrally Acting Muscle Relaxants – Work on the brain and spinal cord.
2. Direct-Acting Muscle Relaxants – Work directly on muscles.

Centrally Acting Muscle Relaxants: Reducing Spasticity via the CNS

These drugs don't work directly on muscles—instead, they slow down nerve signals in the brain and spinal cord, helping muscles relax.

Common Centrally Acting Muscle Relaxants

- Carisoprodol
- Cyclobenzaprine (longest duration: 12–25 hours)
- Methocarbamol
- Metaxalone
- Tizanidine

How These Drugs Work (Pharmacodynamics)

- They act as central nervous system (CNS) depressants.

- They reduce muscle tightness by causing mild sedation and relaxation.
- They don't directly affect muscle contraction or nerve conduction.

How They Move Through the Body (Pharmacokinetics)

- Absorbed through the digestive system.
- Distributed throughout the body and metabolized in the liver.
- Excreted by the kidneys.

Cyclobenzaprine lasts the longest (12 to 25 hours), while other muscle relaxants typically last 4 to 6 hours.

When Are These Drugs Used? (Pharmacotherapeutics)

These medications are prescribed along with rest and physical therapy to relieve:

- Acute muscle pain and spasms.
- Spasticity in conditions like multiple sclerosis and cerebral palsy.

Drug Interactions: What to Avoid

Caution: These drugs interact with other CNS depressants and can cause excessive sedation or breathing problems.

- Alcohol, opioids, and barbiturates – Cause extreme drowsiness.
- Tricyclic antidepressants – May cause dangerous sedation or seizures.
- Antihypertensive drugs – Some muscle relaxants reduce blood pressure, increasing dizziness.
- Hormonal contraceptives – Can slow the clearance of tizanidine, requiring a lower dose.

Side Effects of Muscle Relaxants

Common side effects include:

- Dizziness and drowsiness.
- Nausea, constipation, or diarrhea.

- Heartburn or upset stomach.

Serious Reactions:

- Allergic reactions (rash, swelling, difficulty breathing).
- Heart issues (irregular heartbeat or very low blood pressure).

Long-term use can lead to physical dependence. Stopping suddenly may cause withdrawal symptoms like headaches, nausea, and insomnia.

Nursing Considerations for Muscle Relaxants

1. Assessment: Checking the Patient's Condition

- Monitor muscle pain and spasms regularly.
- Check for allergic reactions or excessive sedation.
- Assess blood pressure to avoid dizziness or fainting.

2. Key Nursing Diagnoses

- Risk for falls due to dizziness.
- Risk for injury due to muscle weakness.
- Deficient knowledge of proper medication use.

3. Implementation: Safe Administration

- Give with food or milk to prevent stomach upset.
- Start with a low dose to reduce side effects.
- Encourage patients to avoid alcohol while taking these medications.

Direct-Acting Muscle Relaxants: Working Directly on Muscles

Unlike centrally acting relaxants, direct-acting muscle relaxants work directly on muscle tissue by blocking calcium release, reducing contraction strength.

The main direct-acting skeletal muscle relaxant is:

- Dantrolene sodium – Used for severe spasticity and malignant hyperthermia (a rare but deadly reaction to anesthesia).

How Dantrolene Works (Pharmacodynamics)

- Reduces muscle contraction by preventing calcium release.
- Doesn't affect the heart or intestines.

When Is Dantrolene Used?

- Cerebral palsy
- Multiple sclerosis
- Spinal cord injuries
- Stroke-related spasticity
- Malignant hyperthermia (a severe reaction to anesthesia)

High doses can cause liver toxicity – patients must be monitored for liver damage.

Drug Interactions with Dantrolene

- CNS depressants (opioids, sedatives, alcohol) – May increase sedation.
- Estrogen-based contraceptives – Increase the risk of liver damage.
- Verapamil (a heart medication) – May cause serious heart rhythm issues.

Side Effects of Dantrolene

- Drowsiness and dizziness.
- Muscle weakness.
- Liver damage with long-term use.

Serious Reactions:

- Seizures or confusion.
- Severe liver toxicity (must monitor liver function).

Nursing Considerations for Dantrolene

1. Assessment: Monitoring Patient's Health

- Check liver function regularly to prevent toxicity.
- Monitor for muscle weakness to avoid falls.
- Assess breathing, as excessive muscle relaxation can affect lung function.

2. Implementation: Administering the Drug Safely

- Give with meals to prevent stomach irritation.
- Monitor for liver toxicity signs (yellowing skin, dark urine).

No Abrupt Endings: The Importance of Gradual Baclofen Withdrawal

When discontinuing intrathecal baclofen, stopping it too quickly can be dangerous. Patients who experience sudden withdrawal may develop:

- High fever.
- Mental confusion or disorientation.
- Severe muscle rigidity and spasms (rebound spasticity).
- In rare cases, complications like rhabdomyolysis (muscle breakdown), multiple organ failure, or even death.

To avoid these risks, baclofen must be tapered off gradually under medical supervision.

Drug Interactions: What to Watch Out For

While baclofen has relatively few drug interactions, certain medications can increase its effects or cause unexpected side effects:

- Alcohol & Other CNS Depressants – Increase drowsiness, dizziness, and risk of falls.
- Fentanyl (a pain reliever) – Can prolong anesthesia effects, making sedation last longer.
- Lithium Carbonate – May worsen hyperkinesia (excessive movement).

- Tricyclic Antidepressants – Can enhance muscle relaxation when combined with baclofen.

Key Warning: Patients should be cautious when combining baclofen with other sedative medications, as it can intensify drowsiness and impair motor function.

Common Side Effects of Baclofen

Most people tolerate baclofen well, but some side effects may occur, including:

Mild Side Effects:

- Drowsiness & fatigue.
- Dizziness or lightheadedness.
- Nausea & stomach discomfort.
- Headache.

Less Common Side Effects:

- Muscle weakness & low muscle tone (hypotonia).
- Depression or mood changes.
- Confusion or memory issues.

Serious Reactions: Seek medical attention for:

- Severe allergic reactions (rash, swelling, difficulty breathing).
- Extreme drowsiness or loss of consciousness.
- Heart rhythm irregularities or low blood pressure.

Nursing Considerations for Baclofen Therapy

1. Assessment: Monitoring Patient Response

- Evaluate muscle spasms and pain before starting baclofen.
- Monitor for allergic reactions or excessive drowsiness.
- Check blood tests (CBC) to ensure no adverse effects on blood cell counts.

2. Key Nursing Diagnoses

- Risk for injury due to dizziness and muscle weakness.
- Acute pain from underlying muscle conditions.
- Deficient knowledge regarding proper medication use.

3. Implementation: Safe Administration Practices

- Administer with food or milk to prevent stomach upset.
- Monitor seizure-prone patients carefully as baclofen withdrawal can increase seizure risk.
- Do not abruptly stop the medication—taper slowly to prevent severe withdrawal symptoms.

4. Evaluation: Measuring Treatment Success

- Has the patient's muscle spasms improved?
- Are side effects manageable?
- Does the patient and family understand how to use baclofen safely?

3.3. Neuromuscular Blocking Drugs: Temporary Muscle Paralysis for Medical Procedures

Neuromuscular blocking drugs temporarily relax muscles by blocking nerve signals at the neuromuscular junction. They do not relieve pain or cause unconsciousness, so they must be used alongside anesthesia and pain medication.

When Are These Drugs Used?

Neuromuscular blockers are commonly used in medical settings for:

- Surgical procedures – To keep muscles relaxed during operations.
- Ventilation support – To help patients who struggle with breathing on their own.

- Seizure management – To reduce muscle spasms in drug-induced or electroconvulsive therapy (ECT) seizures.

Types of Neuromuscular Blockers

There are two main categories of these drugs:

1. Nondepolarizing Neuromuscular Blockers (Block muscle contraction)

- Atracurium
- Cisatracurium
- Rocuronium
- Vecuronium

2. Depolarizing Neuromuscular Blockers (Cause a brief contraction, then paralysis)

- Succinylcholine (short-acting, commonly used for intubation).

How Neuromuscular Blockers Work (Pharmacodynamics)

- Nondepolarizing drugs block acetylcholine, preventing muscles from contracting.
- Depolarizing drugs act like acetylcholine but stay attached longer, leading to temporary paralysis.

Muscle Paralysis Progression

Neuromuscular blockers follow a specific order of paralysis:

- Eyes, face, and neck muscles relax first.
- Arms, legs, and abdominal muscles lose movement.
- Breathing muscles (diaphragm) become paralyzed.

Warning: Patients remain fully conscious and can feel pain while paralyzed—this is why anesthesia and pain relievers must be used together.

How These Drugs Are Processed in the Body (Pharmacokinetics)

- Not absorbed through the stomach – Must be given IV or IM.
- Fast-acting – Effects begin in seconds to minutes.
- Broken down by enzymes in the liver, kidneys, and plasma.

Medical Uses of Neuromuscular Blockers (Pharmacotherapeutics)

- Intubation – Relaxes muscles for inserting a breathing tube.
- Surgery – Prevents muscle movement during delicate procedures.
- ICU Ventilation – Helps sedated patients breathe through a ventilator.
- Bone & Joint Treatments – Used for realigning fractures or dislocated joints.

Drug Interactions: What to Watch Out For

Certain drugs can make neuromuscular blockers stronger or weaker:

Increases Paralysis:

- Anesthetics & antibiotics (aminoglycosides, clindamycin) – Can enhance muscle relaxation.
- Electrolyte imbalances (low potassium or calcium) – Can increase drug effects.

Reduces Paralysis:

- Anticholinesterase drugs (neostigmine, pyridostigmine) – Reverse paralysis after surgery.
- Seizure medications (carbamazepine, phenytoin) – May weaken the drug's effects.

Side Effects & Risks of Neuromuscular Blockers

While these drugs play a vital role in surgery and ICU care, they come with risks:

Common Side Effects

- Low blood pressure (hypotension).
- Temporary breathing difficulty (apnea).
- Skin rashes or reactions.

Serious Risks

Succinylcholine (short-acting blocker) may cause:

- Severe hyperkalemia (dangerous potassium levels in the blood).
- Malignant hyperthermia (life-threatening fever and muscle rigidity).

Nursing Considerations for Neuromuscular Blockers

1. Assessment: Checking Patient's Status

- Monitor breathing carefully (patients need ventilation support).
- Check for muscle recovery using nerve stimulation tests.
- Assess for allergic reactions or skin changes.

2. Implementation: Administering Safely

- Always give with pain relief and sedation (patients can feel pain while paralyzed).
- Monitor vital signs closely to prevent dangerous drops in blood pressure.
- Keep emergency respiratory equipment ready.

3. Evaluation: Ensuring Safe Recovery

- Is the patient breathing normally after the drug wears off?
- Are there signs of muscle recovery?
- Does the patient show any lingering side effects?

3.4. Antiparkinsonian Drugs: Restoring Balance and Movement

Parkinson's disease is a progressive neurological disorder that affects movement and coordination. It is characterized by four key symptoms:

- Muscle rigidity (stiffness and inflexibility).
- Akinesia (difficulty initiating voluntary movements).
- Resting tremors (shaking when muscles are at rest).
- Postural instability (balance and coordination problems).

What Causes Parkinson's Disease?

The brain maintains movement control through a delicate balance of two neurotransmitters:

- Dopamine – A chemical that controls smooth and coordinated movement.
- Acetylcholine – A neurotransmitter that excites muscle activity.

In Parkinson's disease, dopamine-producing nerve cells in the brain gradually degenerate. This reduces dopamine levels, leading to excess acetylcholine, which causes tremors, stiffness, and movement difficulties.

Goals of Parkinson's Drug Therapy

The aim of treatment is to relieve symptoms, improve mobility, and maintain independence. Medications achieve this by:

- Blocking excess acetylcholine (anticholinergic drugs).
- Boosting dopamine levels (dopaminergic drugs).
- Slowing the breakdown of dopamine (COMT inhibitors).

Anticholinergic Drugs: Balancing Neurotransmitters

Anticholinergic drugs block acetylcholine to reduce tremors and muscle stiffness. They are most effective in early-stage Parkinson's disease or when tremors are the primary symptom.

Common Anticholinergic Medications

- Benztropine
- Trihexyphenidyl
- Procyclidine

How They Work (Pharmacodynamics)

- Too much acetylcholine overstimulates movement, causing tremors.
- Anticholinergic drugs block acetylcholine receptors, reducing muscle stiffness and excessive movement.

How These Drugs Are Processed (Pharmacokinetics)

- Well absorbed from the digestive system.
- Cross the blood-brain barrier to act directly on the brain.
- Metabolized in the liver and excreted by the kidneys.

Benztropine has a long duration of action, lasting up to 24 hours in some patients.

When Are These Drugs Used? (Pharmacotherapeutics)

Anticholinergic drugs are most effective in:

- Early Parkinson's disease (when symptoms are mild).
- Tremor-dominant Parkinson's.
- Reducing excessive saliva production (sialorrhea).

However, they are NOT as effective for stiffness and slowness of movement.

Drug Interactions: What to Avoid

Caution: These drugs interact with other medications, increasing side effects.

- Amantadine – May increase unwanted side effects.
- Levodopa – Can reduce absorption, worsening symptoms.
- Antipsychotic medications (haloperidol, phenothiazines) – May make both drugs less effective.
- Over-the-counter cold medicines and diet pills – Can worsen anticholinergic side effects.
- Alcohol – Increases sedation and confusion.

Side Effects of Anticholinergic Drugs

Common Side Effects:

- Dry mouth
- Blurred vision & pupil dilation
- Constipation & nausea
- Urine retention
- Increased heart rate (tachycardia)

Serious Risks (especially in elderly patients):

- Confusion & agitation
- Hallucinations or psychosis-like symptoms
- Increased intraocular pressure (dangerous for glaucoma patients)

Nursing Considerations for Anticholinergic Drugs

1. Assessment: Monitoring the Patient

- Check motor symptoms to determine if the drug is effective.
- Monitor for confusion, drowsiness, or hallucinations.
- Assess urinary function and watch for retention.

2. Key Nursing Diagnoses

- Risk for injury due to confusion or dizziness.
- Impaired physical mobility due to Parkinson's symptoms.
- Deficient knowledge of proper medication use.

3. Implementation: Ensuring Safe Administration

- Give with food to prevent stomach irritation.
- Taper off slowly—never stop suddenly, as symptoms can worsen.
- Encourage hydration and fiber intake to prevent constipation.

4. Evaluation: Measuring Treatment Success

- Has tremor and muscle stiffness improved?

- Are side effects manageable?
- Does the patient understand how to take the medication safely?

Dopaminergic Drugs: Boosting Dopamine to Restore Movement

Dopaminergic drugs increase dopamine levels or mimic its effects in the brain. They are the most effective treatment for Parkinson's disease.

Common Dopaminergic Medications

- Levodopa (converted to dopamine in the brain).
- Carbidopa-Levodopa (Sinemet) – a combination that improves levodopa's effectiveness.
- Amantadine – an antiviral drug that increases dopamine release.
- Ropinirole & Pramipexole – dopamine receptor stimulators (agonists).
- Selegiline – slows the breakdown of dopamine.

How These Drugs Work (Pharmacodynamics)

- Levodopa is converted into dopamine, replenishing brain levels.
- Carbidopa prevents levodopa breakdown before it reaches the brain.
- Dopamine agonists (Ropinirole, Pramipexole) directly stimulate dopamine receptors.

How These Drugs Are Processed (Pharmacokinetics)

- Absorbed through the digestive system.
- Metabolized in the liver or kidneys.
- Eliminated through urine and feces.

Levodopa absorption is reduced when taken with protein-rich foods.

When Are These Drugs Used? (Pharmacotherapeutics)

- Levodopa is the most effective treatment for Parkinson's disease.

- Dopamine agonists (Ropinirole, Pramipexole) are used in early or mild cases.
- Selegiline extends the effect of levodopa.

Drug Interactions: What to Avoid

Levodopa can interact with many medications, leading to dangerous effects:

- MAO inhibitors (tranylcypromine, phenelzine) – May cause severe high blood pressure.
- Vitamin B6 (pyridoxine) – Reduces the effectiveness of levodopa.
- Antipsychotic medications – May block dopamine and worsen symptoms.

Side Effects of Dopaminergic Drugs

Common Side Effects:

- Nausea & vomiting
- Dizziness & low blood pressure (orthostatic hypotension)
- Confusion & hallucinations

Serious Risks:

- Levodopa may cause abnormal movements (dyskinesia).
- Sudden "on-off" episodes – periods of good movement followed by stiffness.
- Stopping these drugs too quickly may cause a severe withdrawal reaction (neuroleptic malignant syndrome).

Nursing Considerations for Dopaminergic Drugs

1. Assessment: Monitoring for Effectiveness

- Check for improvement in movement and tremors.
- Monitor blood pressure for dizziness or fainting.
- Watch for signs of excessive movements (dyskinesia).

- Take levodopa on an empty stomach (or with low-protein food).
- Adjust dosage gradually to avoid side effects.
- Monitor for sudden worsening of symptoms ("on-off" effect).

3.5. Anticonvulsant Drugs: Controlling Seizures and Protecting Brain Function

Anticonvulsant drugs play a crucial role in managing seizures and epilepsy by stabilizing nerve activity in the brain. These medications help:

- Prevent recurrent seizures in people with chronic epilepsy.
- Control sudden seizures caused by brain injuries or surgery.
- Treat status epilepticus, a life-threatening condition of continuous seizures.

How Anticonvulsants Work

Seizures occur when nerve cells in the brain fire abnormally and excessively, disrupting normal function. Anticonvulsants help by:

- Blocking nerve overactivity to prevent seizures from starting.
- Slowing down electrical signals in the brain.
- Altering neurotransmitters (chemical messengers) to calm nerve impulses.

Important:

- Treatment usually begins with ONE drug and the dosage is increased gradually.
- If the first drug isn't effective, another single drug is tried before adding combination therapy.

Types of Anticonvulsants

Anticonvulsants are divided into several classes based on how they work:

1. Hydantoins (e.g., phenytoin, fosphenytoin) – Block excessive nerve activity.
2. Barbiturates (e.g., phenobarbital, primidone) – Calm brain activity.
3. Iminostilbenes (e.g., carbamazepine) – Reduce nerve firing.
4. Benzodiazepines (e.g., diazepam, lorazepam) – Act as sedatives to stop seizures quickly.
5. Carboxylic acid derivatives (e.g., valproic acid) – Increase calming neurotransmitters.
6. Others – Includes newer drugs like lamotrigine, gabapentin, and levetiracetam.

Hydantoins: The Most Commonly Used Anticonvulsants

Common Hydantoins:

- Phenytoin (Dilantin) – The most widely used anticonvulsant.
- Fosphenytoin – A short-term IV/IM version of phenytoin.
- Ethotoin – Used when other drugs are not tolerated.

How Hydantoins Work (Pharmacodynamics)

- Stabilize nerve cells in the brain to prevent excessive firing.
- Slow the spread of seizure activity across the brain.
- Work mainly in the motor cortex, where movement control is affected by seizures.

How These Drugs Are Processed (Pharmacokinetics)

- Phenytoin is absorbed slowly but spreads quickly throughout the body.
- Highly protein-bound (90%), meaning only a small portion is active at a time.

- Metabolized in the liver and excreted in urine.

Dosing Note:

Phenytoin metabolism is not linear—small dosage changes can lead to big shifts in drug levels, increasing the risk of toxicity.

Therapeutic blood level: 10–20 mcg/mL.

When Are Hydantoins Used? (Pharmacotherapeutics)

- Partial seizures (affecting one part of the brain).
- Tonic-clonic seizures (full-body convulsions).
- Status epilepticus (given IV after benzodiazepines to maintain seizure control).

Ethotoin may be combined with other anticonvulsants if phenytoin alone isn't effective.

Drug Interactions: What to Watch Out For

Drugs That Reduce Phenytoin's Effectiveness:

- Phenobarbital, theophylline, carbamazepine, rifampin – Can lower phenytoin levels, making it less effective.
- Antacids & tube feedings – Decrease absorption (stop tube feedings 2 hours before & after phenytoin).

Drugs That Increase Phenytoin's Effects (Risk of Toxicity!):

- Valproic acid, cimetidine, fluconazole, amiodarone – Can increase phenytoin levels and cause toxicity.
- Warfarin & hormonal contraceptives – Phenytoin reduces their effectiveness, increasing the risk of pregnancy or blood clots.

Side Effects & Risks of Hydantoins

Common Side Effects:

- Drowsiness, dizziness, and fatigue.
- Nausea, vomiting, and stomach pain.

- Gum overgrowth (gingival hyperplasia) – Requires good oral hygiene.

Serious Risks:

- Irregular heartbeat (arrhythmia) – Seen with IV administration.
- Liver damage – Requires periodic liver function tests.
- Severe skin reactions (Stevens-Johnson syndrome).

Nursing Considerations for Hydantoins

1. Assessment: Monitoring the Patient

- Check serum drug levels (10–20 mcg/mL) to avoid toxicity.
- Monitor for allergic reactions and skin rashes.
- Assess liver function and complete blood count (CBC) every 6 months.

2. Key Nursing Diagnoses

- Risk for injury due to dizziness or drowsiness.
- Impaired physical mobility due to sedation.
- Noncompliance risk due to long-term therapy requirements.

3. Implementation: Safe Administration

- Give with food to prevent stomach irritation.
- Avoid IV administration in small veins (prevents purple glove syndrome).
- Dilute IV phenytoin with normal saline and infuse over 30–60 minutes.

4. Evaluation: Measuring Treatment Success

- Are seizures under control?
- Is the patient tolerating the drug without major side effects?
- Does the patient understand how to take the medication safely?

Barbiturates: Less Common But Still Effective

Phenobarbital, once a first-line seizure treatment, is now used only when other drugs fail because it causes significant sedation.

When Are Barbiturates Used?

- Partial seizures & tonic-clonic seizures (alternative treatment).
- Status epilepticus (IV use if other drugs don't work).
- Febrile seizures in children (rare cases).

Phenobarbital has a delayed onset when used IV, making it less ideal for emergency seizures.

Side Effects of Barbiturates

Common Side Effects:

- Drowsiness, dizziness, and lethargy.
- Depression & memory problems (especially in older adults).

Serious Risks:

- Breathing problems & laryngospasm (when given IV).
- Low blood pressure.
- Physical dependence with long-term use.

Administering Anticonvulsants Safely: Avoiding Risks & Ensuring Effectiveness

1. Injection Safety Matters

- IM injections must be given deep into muscle tissue. A shallow injection can cause pain, tissue damage, and abscess formation.
- Dosages should be adjusted based on how the patient responds.
- Monitor for central nervous system (CNS) side effects, such as drowsiness, confusion, or dizziness, which can increase the risk of falls or injury.

2. Evaluating Treatment Success

- The patient has no serious side effects or injuries.
- Seizures are well-controlled, and the patient can perform daily activities (ADLs) normally.
- The patient follows the prescribed treatment plan.

Iminostilbenes: A Key Anticonvulsant Option

Carbamazepine is the most widely used drug in this class. It is effective in treating:

- Partial seizures (including simple and complex types).
- Generalized tonic-clonic seizures (affecting the entire brain).
- Mixed seizure types.

How Carbamazepine Works (Pharmacodynamics)

- Prevents excessive nerve activity, stopping the spread of seizures.
- Stabilizes brain cells to reduce abnormal electrical impulses.
- Similar to phenytoin, but with additional pain-relieving properties.

How Carbamazepine Is Processed (Pharmacokinetics)

- Absorbed slowly from the digestive system.
- Metabolized in the liver and excreted through urine.
- Binds to plasma proteins (75-90%), meaning only a portion of the drug remains active at any time.
- Blood levels must be monitored (therapeutic range: 4-12 mcg/mL).

When Is Carbamazepine Used? (Pharmacotherapeutics)

- First-line treatment for tonic-clonic and partial seizures.
- Relieves facial nerve pain (trigeminal neuralgia).
- May be used for bipolar disorder or explosive mood disorders.

Not recommended for absence or myoclonic seizures—it may worsen these conditions.

Drug Interactions: What to Watch For

Carbamazepine can lower the effectiveness of many medications, including:

- Oral contraceptives – Increases the risk of unintended pregnancy.
- Blood thinners (warfarin, anticoagulants) – Reduces their effect, increasing the risk of blood clots.
- Antidepressants (tricyclics, bupropion, SSRIs) – May become less effective.

Drugs That Increase Carbamazepine Levels (Risk of Toxicity!):

- Cimetidine (acid reducer), erythromycin (antibiotic), SSRIs, and ketoconazole (antifungal).

Drugs That Reduce Carbamazepine Levels (Decreasing Effectiveness):

- Phenytoin, barbiturates, and felbamate.

Even certain herbal supplements, like plantain, can interfere with absorption!

Side Effects of Carbamazepine

Common Side Effects:

- Drowsiness & dizziness.
- Nausea, vomiting, or stomach pain.
- Skin rashes (some may indicate a serious allergic reaction).

Serious Risks:

- Rare but dangerous blood disorders (low red or white blood cells).
- Stevens-Johnson Syndrome (a life-threatening skin condition).
- Liver toxicity – Regular liver function tests are required.

Warning for Asian Patients:

- People of Asian descent should be genetically tested before taking carbamazepine due to an increased risk of Stevens-Johnson Syndrome.

Nursing Considerations for Carbamazepine

1. Assessment: Monitoring Patient Response

- Check seizure history and effectiveness of treatment.
- Monitor blood tests regularly (CBC, liver function, and drug levels).
- Assess for skin rashes, unusual bruising, or fatigue, which could indicate serious reactions.

2. Implementation: Safe Administration

- Give with food to reduce stomach irritation.
- Shake liquid suspensions well before measuring a dose.
- Monitor for signs of overdose, such as confusion or unsteady movements.

3. Evaluation: Measuring Treatment Success

- Seizures are well-controlled with minimal side effects.
- The patient follows the medication schedule and understands how to take it properly.
- No severe drug reactions or complications occur.

Benzodiazepines: Quick-Acting Seizure Control

Benzodiazepines are commonly used to stop seizures quickly but are not usually for long-term seizure management.

Common Benzodiazepines Used for Seizures:

- Diazepam (Valium) – Used for emergency seizures & repetitive seizures (rectal form available for children).
- Lorazepam (Ativan) – First-choice drug for status epilepticus (continuous seizures).

- Clonazepam (Klonopin) – Only benzodiazepine used for long-term seizure control.
- Clorazepate – Used as an add-on treatment for partial seizures.

How Benzodiazepines Work (Pharmacodynamics)

- Enhance GABA activity, the brain's natural calming chemical.
- Slow nerve signals, preventing seizure activity.
- Cause sedation and muscle relaxation.

Warning: These drugs are highly sedating and can cause drowsiness, dizziness, and confusion.

How They Are Processed (Pharmacokinetics)

- Absorbed quickly when taken orally or IV.
- Metabolized in the liver and excreted in urine.
- Cross the placenta and appear in breast milk, so caution is needed for pregnant or breastfeeding patients.

When Are Benzodiazepines Used? (Pharmacotherapeutics)

- Status epilepticus (continuous seizures) – Lorazepam is the drug of choice.
- Stopping acute seizures (IV diazepam or lorazepam).
- Long-term seizure prevention (clonazepam for certain types of epilepsy).
- Repetitive seizures (diazepam rectal gel is available for children).

Not used for daily seizure prevention due to high addiction potential.

Drug Interactions: What to Avoid

Drugs That Increase Sedation with Benzodiazepines:

- Opioids, alcohol, sleeping pills, and muscle relaxants.
- Cimetidine and hormonal contraceptives – May cause excessive drowsiness.

Side Effects of Benzodiazepines

Common Side Effects:

- Drowsiness & fatigue.
- Dizziness & poor coordination.
- Weakness & confusion.

Serious Risks:

- Respiratory depression (slowed breathing) – High doses of IV benzodiazepines can be life-threatening.
- Dependence & withdrawal symptoms if stopped suddenly.

Nursing Considerations for Benzodiazepines

1. Assessment: Monitoring for Safety

- Check respiratory rate every 5-15 minutes for IV use.
- Monitor liver and kidney function with long-term use.
- Watch for overdose symptoms (extreme drowsiness, confusion, slow breathing).

2. Implementation: Safe Administration

- Give oral doses with food to reduce stomach irritation.
- For IV diazepam, administer slowly (5 mg/min) and have resuscitation equipment ready.
- Limit rectal diazepam to no more than five episodes per month.

3. Evaluation: Measuring Treatment Success

- Seizures are controlled without excessive sedation.
- The patient understands the risks of dependence.
- No serious breathing complications occur.

Gabapentin: A Versatile Anticonvulsant and Nerve Pain Reliever

Gabapentin is a widely used anticonvulsant that was originally designed to mimic the neurotransmitter GABA (gamma-aminobutyric acid). However, its exact mechanism of action remains unclear.

Aside from treating partial seizures, gabapentin is also used for:

- Nerve pain caused by diabetes (diabetic neuropathy) and shingles (postherpetic neuralgia).
- Multiple sclerosis tremors.
- Bipolar disorder.
- Migraine prevention.
- Parkinson's disease symptoms.

How Gabapentin Works (Pharmacodynamics)

- Does NOT directly affect GABA receptors as originally intended.
- Binds to a special protein in the brain, possibly increasing GABA levels indirectly.
- Calms overactive nerve signals, making it useful for seizures and chronic nerve pain.

How Gabapentin Is Processed (Pharmacokinetics)

- Absorbed in the digestive system (but absorption decreases at higher doses).
- NOT metabolized by the liver, meaning it does not affect liver enzymes.
- Excreted entirely by the kidneys, so patients with kidney disease need lower doses.

When Is Gabapentin Used? (Pharmacotherapeutics)

- Adjunct therapy for partial seizures (ages 3 and older).
- Neuropathic pain (diabetic nerve pain, shingles pain).

72

- Migraine prevention and MS tremors.
- Mood stabilization in bipolar disorder (off-label use).

Not recommended for myoclonic seizures—it may worsen them.

Drug Interactions: What to Watch Out For

Drugs That Affect Gabapentin:

- Antacids (e.g., Tums, Maalox) – Reduce gabapentin absorption.
- Cimetidine (heartburn medication) – Can alter gabapentin levels.

Take gabapentin at least 2 hours after taking an antacid.

Side Effects of Gabapentin

Common Side Effects:

- Fatigue & drowsiness.
- Dizziness & loss of coordination (ataxia).
- Mild nausea & stomach upset.

Less Common But Serious Reactions:

- Swelling (edema), weight gain.
- Mood changes, aggression, or emotional instability.
- Blurred vision & eye twitching (nystagmus, diplopia).
- Respiratory issues (bronchitis, shortness of breath).

Sudden withdrawal can trigger seizures—dose must be tapered gradually!

Nursing Considerations for Gabapentin

1. Assessment: Monitoring Patient Response

- Check seizure history and frequency of nerve pain.
- Monitor kidney function, especially in elderly patients.
- Assess for mood changes, as gabapentin can affect emotions.

2. Implementation: Safe Administration

- Give with food to prevent stomach irritation.
- Start the first dose at bedtime to reduce dizziness.
- Slowly decrease dose over a week if stopping the drug—never stop abruptly!

3. Evaluation: Measuring Treatment Success

- Seizures or nerve pain are well-controlled.
- The patient can tolerate side effects without major issues.
- The patient follows the prescribed dosage schedule.

Lamotrigine: A Flexible Anticonvulsant with Mood Benefits

Lamotrigine is an anticonvulsant approved for epilepsy and bipolar disorder. It works by blocking sodium channels in nerve cells, reducing excessive brain activity that leads to seizures and mood instability.

When Is Lamotrigine Used? (Pharmacotherapeutics)

- Partial & generalized seizures (including Lennox-Gastaut syndrome).
- Bipolar disorder (helps stabilize mood swings).
- Alternative to other seizure medications that cause excessive sedation.

Can worsen myoclonic seizures in some patients.

How Lamotrigine Works (Pharmacodynamics)

- Blocks sodium channels, preventing nerve overactivity.
- Reduces the release of excitatory neurotransmitters (glutamate, aspartate).
- Improves mood in bipolar patients by stabilizing brain activity.

How Lamotrigine Is Processed (Pharmacokinetics)

- Well absorbed in the digestive system.

- Metabolized in the liver and excreted by the kidneys.
- Clearance is affected by other seizure medications.

If taken with valproic acid, clearance is reduced—dose adjustments are needed!

Drug Interactions: What to Avoid

Drugs That Lower Lamotrigine Levels (Making It Less Effective):

- Carbamazepine, phenytoin, phenobarbital.
- Acetaminophen (Tylenol) in high doses.

Drugs That Increase Lamotrigine Levels (Risk of Toxicity!):

- Valproic acid (requires a lower lamotrigine dose).
- Folate inhibitors (can cause additive effects).

Side Effects of Lamotrigine

Common Side Effects:

- Dizziness, headache, drowsiness.
- Double vision (diplopia), nausea.

Serious Risk: Stevens-Johnson Syndrome (SJS)

- A potentially life-threatening rash that can occur within 3–4 weeks of starting the drug.
- Black Box Warning: If a rash develops, stop the medication immediately!
- Starting at high doses or increasing too quickly raises the risk.

Nursing Considerations for Lamotrigine

1. Assessment: Monitoring Patient Safety

- Monitor for early signs of rash or skin reactions.
- Check seizure frequency and severity.
- Assess mood in bipolar patients for improvement or worsening symptoms.

2. Implementation: Safe Administration

- Give with food to minimize stomach irritation.
- Start at a low dose and increase gradually to prevent serious rash.
- Never stop abruptly—withdraw over at least 2 weeks.

3. Evaluation: Measuring Treatment Success

- Seizures are under control without major side effects.
- No rash or severe allergic reactions develop.
- Bipolar patients experience improved mood stability.

Oxcarbazepine: A Safer Alternative to Carbamazepine

Oxcarbazepine is chemically similar to carbamazepine but with fewer liver interactions.

When Is Oxcarbazepine Used? (Pharmacotherapeutics)

- Partial seizures (as monotherapy or adjunctive therapy).
- Alternative for patients who cannot tolerate carbamazepine.

May worsen absence or myoclonic seizures.

How Oxcarbazepine Works (Pharmacodynamics)

- Blocks sodium channels, reducing seizure spread.
- Prevents excessive electrical activity in the brain.

How Oxcarbazepine Is Processed (Pharmacokinetics)

- Absorbed completely in the digestive system.
- Metabolized into its active form (MHD) in the liver.
- Excreted primarily by the kidneys.

Unlike carbamazepine, oxcarbazepine does NOT induce its own metabolism.

Drug Interactions: What to Watch Out For

Drugs That Lower Oxcarbazepine Levels:

- Carbamazepine, phenytoin, valproic acid, phenobarbital.

Oxcarbazepine Can Reduce the Effectiveness Of:

- Birth control pills (increases pregnancy risk!).
- Calcium channel blockers (e.g., verapamil).
- Side Effects of Oxcarbazepine

Common Side Effects:

- Drowsiness, dizziness, blurred vision.
- Nausea, vomiting, upset stomach.

Serious Risk: Hyponatremia (Low Sodium Levels)

- Can cause confusion, seizures, or weakness—monitor sodium levels.

Nursing Considerations for Oxcarbazepine

- Monitor for allergic reactions (especially in patients allergic to carbamazepine).
- Check sodium levels regularly.
- Taper dose gradually to avoid seizure rebound.

Ensuring Safe Administration of Anticonvulsants

Shaking Things Up: Proper Use of Oral Suspensions

- Shake well before use to ensure an even mixture of medication.
- Can be mixed with water or taken directly from the syringe.
- Can be taken with or without food.
- Oral suspension and tablet doses are interchangeable at the same strength.

Adjusting Treatment for the Best Outcome

- Dosage may need adjustments based on the patient's response.

- Monitor for central nervous system (CNS) side effects, such as drowsiness or dizziness.

Evaluating Treatment Success

- Patient remains free from injury related to medication effects.
- Patient maintains mobility and daily activity levels.
- Patient follows prescribed treatment and remains seizure-free.

Topiramate: A Unique Anticonvulsant for Seizures and More

Topiramate belongs to a distinct class of anticonvulsants that work differently from other seizure medications. Instead of raising the seizure threshold, it prevents seizures from spreading in the brain.

When Is Topiramate Used? (Pharmacotherapeutics)

- Adjunct therapy for partial and generalized tonic-clonic seizures (ages 2 and older).
- Lennox-Gastaut syndrome (a severe childhood epilepsy).
- May also be effective as a stand-alone (monotherapy) seizure treatment.

May be useful for other seizure types but requires further study.

How Topiramate Works (Pharmacodynamics)

- Blocks voltage-dependent sodium channels, reducing nerve overactivity.
- Enhances GABA receptor activity, increasing the brain's natural calming effects.
- Blocks glutamate receptors, preventing excessive nerve stimulation.

How Topiramate Is Processed (Pharmacokinetics)

- Rapidly absorbed in the digestive system.
- Partially metabolized in the liver.

- Mostly excreted unchanged in the urine.

Patients with kidney disease require lower doses, and those on dialysis may need extra doses to compensate for drug loss during treatment.

Drug Interactions: What to Watch For

Drugs That Lower Topiramate Levels (Making It Less Effective):

- Carbamazepine, phenytoin, valproic acid (other seizure medications).

Topiramate Can Lower the Effectiveness Of:

- Hormonal contraceptives (birth control) – Increases pregnancy risk!
- Valproic acid – Can reduce drug levels, requiring dose adjustments.

Side Effects of Topiramate

Common Side Effects:

- Drowsiness, dizziness, and headaches.
- Nervousness, confusion, and difficulty concentrating.
- Tingling in hands or feet (paresthesia).

Less Common But Serious Side Effects:

- Liver failure.
- Heatstroke and decreased sweating (hypohidrosis).
- Kidney stones (renal calculi) – Patients should increase fluid intake.

Cognitive side effects (difficulty finding words, memory problems) may require stopping the drug.

Nursing Considerations for Topiramate

1. Assessment: Monitoring Patient Safety

- Monitor seizure frequency and severity.
- Assess mental function for memory issues or cognitive slowing.

- Check for heat intolerance, especially in summer (risk of heatstroke).

2. Implementation: Safe Administration

- Give with food to prevent stomach irritation.
- Adjust doses gradually to minimize cognitive side effects.
- If kidney disease is present, reduce dosage.

3. Evaluation: Measuring Treatment Success

- Seizures are well-controlled with minimal side effects.
- Patient maintains normal mental function.
- No serious adverse reactions occur.

Ethosuximide: The Primary Drug for Absence Seizures

Ethosuximide is a first-choice medication for absence seizures (formerly called "petit mal" seizures).

How Ethosuximide Works (Pharmacodynamics)

- Raises the seizure threshold, making seizures less likely.
- Suppresses abnormal electrical activity in the motor cortex and basal ganglia.

How Ethosuximide Is Processed (Pharmacokinetics)

- Absorbed well from the digestive system.
- Metabolized in the liver and excreted in the urine.
- Long elimination half-life:
  60 hours in adults.
  30 hours in children (so they need more frequent dosing).

When Is Ethosuximide Used? (Pharmacotherapeutics)

- First-line treatment for absence seizures.
- May be combined with valproic acid for difficult-to-control absence seizures.

Not effective for tonic-clonic or partial seizures.

Drug Interactions: What to Watch For

May interact with other seizure medications:

- Can raise phenytoin (Dilantin) levels, increasing toxicity risk.
- Carbamazepine (Tegretol) may speed up ethosuximide metabolism, reducing its effectiveness.
- Valproic acid may either increase or decrease ethosuximide levels.

Side Effects of Ethosuximide

Common Side Effects:

- Nausea, vomiting, and stomach pain (in up to 40% of patients).
- Drowsiness, dizziness, and lethargy.
- Hiccups and headaches.

Rare But Serious Side Effects:

- Blood disorders (low white blood cells, platelets, or red blood cells).
- Severe skin reactions (Stevens-Johnson Syndrome, lupus-like syndrome).
- Psychotic behavior or mood changes.

Patients should report unexplained rashes or mood changes immediately.

Nursing Considerations for Ethosuximide

1. Assessment: Monitoring Patient Safety

- Monitor seizure control and medication blood levels.
- Check for side effects, especially stomach discomfort or rashes.
- Assess emotional well-being, as mood changes can occur.

2. Implementation: Safe Administration

- Give with food to prevent stomach irritation.

- Adjust doses based on seizure control and side effects.

3. Evaluation: Measuring Treatment Success

- Absence seizures are well-controlled.
- Patient tolerates medication without serious side effects.
- Patient remains compliant with therapy.

Zonisamide: A Sulfonamide-Based Anticonvulsant

- Zonisamide is a sulfonamide drug approved for partial seizure treatment in adults.
- Patients allergic to sulfa drugs should not take zonisamide!

When Is Zonisamide Used? (Pharmacotherapeutics)

- Adjunct therapy for partial seizures.
- May also help with myoclonic, generalized, and absence seizures (off-label use).

How Zonisamide Works (Pharmacodynamics)

- Stabilizes nerve membranes to reduce excessive activity.
- Prevents abnormal neuron firing to stop seizures.

How Zonisamide Is Processed (Pharmacokinetics)

- Reaches peak levels in 2–6 hours.
- Metabolized in the liver (CYP3A4 enzyme).
- Excreted in urine as a metabolite.

Older adults may need lower doses due to kidney function decline.

Drug Interactions: What to Watch For

Drugs That Reduce Zonisamide Levels (Less Effective):

- Phenytoin, carbamazepine, phenobarbital.

Serious Side Effects:

- Stevens-Johnson Syndrome (life-threatening rash).
- Psychosis & hallucinations.
- Aplastic anemia (dangerously low blood cells).
- Decreased sweating & risk of heatstroke (especially in children).

Patients should drink plenty of fluids to prevent kidney stones.

Nursing Considerations for Zonisamide

- Monitor for allergic reactions, especially in sulfa-sensitive patients.
- Ensure proper hydration to avoid kidney stones.
- Monitor body temperature in hot weather (risk of heatstroke).

3.6. Antimigraine Medications: Understanding Treatment Options

Migraines are recurring headache disorders that affect millions of people worldwide. They are typically described as a throbbing or pounding headache, often on one side of the head, and may be accompanied by:

- Sensitivity to light and sound.
- Nausea and vomiting.
- Digestive issues (constipation or diarrhea).
- An aura (visual disturbances, tingling, or numbness) before the headache begins.

Migraines are believed to be caused by abnormal blood vessel dilation and inflammation in the brain's trigeminal nerve system.

Migraine Treatment: Stopping an Attack vs. Preventing It

Migraine treatment falls into two categories:

1. Abortive (Symptomatic) Treatment – Stops a migraine once it starts.

2. Preventative (Prophylactic) Treatment – Reduces how often and how severely migraines occur.

Abortive Treatments Include:

- Pain relievers (Aspirin, Acetaminophen, NSAIDs like Ibuprofen or Naproxen).
- Ergotamine derivatives (used less often today).
- 5-HT Agonists (Triptans) – The first-choice drugs for moderate to severe migraines.

Preventative Treatments Include:

- Beta-blockers (e.g., propranolol, metoprolol).
- Tricyclic antidepressants (e.g., amitriptyline).
- Antiseizure medications (e.g., valproic acid, topiramate).
- NSAIDs (for frequent menstrual migraines).

Triptans: The First-Choice Migraine Medications

Triptans are serotonin receptor agonists that help stop migraines in progress.

Common Triptan Medications Include:

- Sumatriptan (available as a pill, nasal spray, or injection).
- Rizatriptan (available as a dissolvable tablet).
- Zolmitriptan.
- Almotriptan.
- Eletriptan.
- Frovatriptan (longest duration, best for recurrent migraines).
- Naratriptan.

Triptans are NOT painkillers! Instead, they constrict blood vessels and reduce inflammation in the brain to stop a migraine attack.

How Triptans Work (Pharmacodynamics)

- Activate serotonin (5-HT1) receptors, which narrow blood vessels in the brain.
- Block inflammatory signals in the trigeminal nerve, reducing pain.
- Relieve migraine symptoms (headache, nausea, and light sensitivity).

How Triptans Are Processed (Pharmacokinetics)

- Most triptans have a half-life of about 2 hours.
- Frovatriptan lasts the longest (25 hours) but takes longer to start working.
- Sumatriptan injection works the fastest (best for severe attacks).

Triptans work best when taken at the first sign of a migraine.

Choosing the Right Triptan

Patients who get nausea and vomiting with migraines may prefer:

- Sumatriptan nasal spray or injection (works fast and bypasses the stomach).
- Rizatriptan dissolvable tablet (no swallowing needed).

Patients with recurrent migraines may need longer-lasting triptans:

- Frovatriptan or Naratriptan – These last longer but take longer to start working.

Patients who want rapid relief may prefer:

- Eletriptan or Almotriptan – Faster onset than some other triptans.

Who Should NOT Take Triptans? (Contraindications)

Triptans should NOT be used by people with:

- Heart disease or high blood pressure (triptans constrict blood vessels).
- Stroke or history of mini-strokes (TIAs).
- Hemiplegic or basilar migraines.
- Severe liver or kidney disease.

Triptan Drug Interactions: What to Avoid

Do NOT take Triptans within 24 hours of these drugs:

- Another triptan or ergotamine – Can cause dangerous blood vessel spasms.
- Dihydroergotamine (another migraine medication) – Increases vasoconstriction risk.

Avoid Eletriptan within 72 hours of:

- CYP3A4 inhibitors (ketoconazole, clarithromycin, ritonavir, etc.) – Can dangerously increase triptan levels.

Avoid triptans with these antidepressants due to serotonin syndrome risk:

- SSRIs (fluoxetine, sertraline, etc.).
- MAO inhibitors (phenelzine, isocarboxazid, etc.).

Frovatriptan levels may be 30% higher in women taking birth control pills.

Side Effects of Triptans

Common Side Effects:

- Tingling, flushing, warmth.
- Dizziness & drowsiness.
- Neck, jaw, or chest tightness (usually harmless but should be monitored).

Serious Risks (Rare):

- Heart attack or irregular heartbeat (higher risk in heart patients).

- Serotonin syndrome (if combined with SSRIs or MAOIs).

Nursing Considerations for Triptans

1. Assessment: Monitoring Patient Safety

- Check for heart disease, high blood pressure, or stroke history before prescribing.
- Monitor ECG in patients at risk for heart disease.
- Ask about past migraine treatments to prevent interactions.

2. Implementation: Safe Administration

- Take as soon as migraine symptoms appear.
- If the migraine returns, a second dose may be taken after 2 hours (but no more than 2 doses in 24 hours).
- Reduce dosage for patients with kidney or liver disease.

3. Evaluation: Measuring Treatment Success

- Migraine symptoms improve, and pain is reduced.
- No serious side effects occur.
- Patient understands how to use the medication safely.

Ergotamine: An Older But Effective Migraine Treatment

Ergotamine was one of the first migraine treatments but is now used less often due to triptans being safer and more effective.

Common Ergotamine Medications:

- Ergotamine (oral, sublingual, or rectal) – Often combined with caffeine.
- Dihydroergotamine (DHE-45, Migranal) – Available as an injection or nasal spray.

Ergotamine should NOT be taken within 24 hours of a triptan!

How Ergotamine Works (Pharmacodynamics)

- Reduces neurogenic inflammation that triggers migraines.
- Constricts blood vessels in the brain.

Dihydroergotamine is preferred over ergotamine because it causes less nausea and fewer side effects.

Side Effects of Ergotamine

Common Side Effects:

- Nausea and vomiting.
- Tingling, numbness, or muscle pain.
- Cold hands and feet (vasoconstriction effect).

Serious Risks (Rare but Dangerous):

- Severe vasoconstriction (leading to gangrene or stroke).
- Rebound headaches if overused.

Patients on beta-blockers (e.g., propranolol) should use ergotamine with caution due to increased vasoconstriction risk.

Chapter 4: Pain Medications

4.1. Understanding Pain Medications: From Mild Relief to Potent Treatments

Pain management medications range from simple over-the-counter (OTC) pain relievers to powerful prescription drugs, including anesthetics. These medications fall into three main categories:

- Nonopioid analgesics, antipyretics, and NSAIDs (pain relievers and fever reducers).
- Opioid analgesics (strong painkillers that act on the nervous system).
- Anesthetic drugs (used for pain relief during surgery or medical procedures).

4.2. Nonopioid Pain Relievers: Safe and Effective for Mild to Moderate Pain

Nonopioid pain relievers help manage pain and fever and reduce inflammation. They do NOT cause dependence, making them safer for long-term use.

Types of Nonopioid Pain Relievers:

- Salicylates (Aspirin) – A common pain reliever with anti-inflammatory and blood-thinning properties.
- Acetaminophen (Tylenol) – A popular pain and fever reducer without anti-inflammatory effects.
- NSAIDs (Ibuprofen, Naproxen, Celecoxib) – Reduce pain, fever, and inflammation.
- Phenazopyridine – A urinary tract analgesic used for UTI pain relief.

Aspirin and Salicylates: A Common and Cost-Effective Option

Aspirin and other salicylates are widely used for pain relief, fever reduction, and inflammation control.

Why Salicylates Are Popular:

- Inexpensive and available without a prescription.
- Effective for conditions like arthritis and muscle pain.
- Aspirin helps prevent heart attacks and strokes by reducing blood clots.

How Aspirin Works (Pharmacodynamics)

- Blocks prostaglandins – chemicals that cause pain and inflammation.
- Reduces fever by stimulating heat loss in the body.
- Prevents blood clots by stopping platelet aggregation (helps prevent heart attacks and strokes).

NSAIDs also block prostaglandins, but aspirin's blood-thinning effects last longer.

How Aspirin Is Processed (Pharmacokinetics)

- Absorbed in the stomach and small intestine.
- Metabolized by the liver into active compounds.
- Excreted by the kidneys.

Enteric-coated aspirin is absorbed more slowly and is better for long-term use (e.g., arthritis) but is not ideal for fast pain relief.

Who Should Use Aspirin? (Pharmacotherapeutics)

- Pain relief (headaches, muscle pain, arthritis, etc.).
- Fever reduction.
- Heart attack and stroke prevention (low-dose aspirin therapy).

Who Should AVOID Aspirin?

- Children under 12 (risk of Reye's syndrome – a rare but serious condition).
- People with ulcers or stomach issues (aspirin can irritate the stomach lining).
- Patients taking blood thinners (increased risk of bleeding).

Aspirin Drug Interactions: What to Watch Out For

Drugs That May Become Stronger (Increased Risk of Side Effects):

- Blood thinners (warfarin, heparin) – Higher risk of bleeding.
- Methotrexate (used for cancer and arthritis) – Increased toxicity.
- Insulin & oral diabetes medications – Higher risk of low blood sugar.

Drugs That May Become Weaker (Reduced Effectiveness):

- Gout medications (probenecid, sulfinpyrazone) – May not work as well.
- Corticosteroids (prednisone, dexamethasone) – Can lower aspirin levels but increase the risk of ulcers.
- Antacids – May reduce aspirin absorption.

Side Effects of Aspirin

Common Side Effects:

- Upset stomach, nausea, and heartburn.
- Increased risk of bleeding (including easy bruising or nosebleeds).

Serious Side Effects (Rare but Dangerous):

- Tinnitus (ringing in the ears) – Can be an early sign of toxicity.
- Stomach ulcers or internal bleeding.
- Reye's syndrome (in children with flu or chickenpox).

Nursing Considerations for Aspirin

1. Assessment: Monitoring Patient Safety

- Check for stomach issues, history of ulcers, or bleeding disorders.
- Monitor for unusual bruising or signs of internal bleeding.
- Ensure patients know to stop aspirin 5–7 days before surgery (to reduce bleeding risk).

2. Implementation: Safe Administration

- Give with food, milk, or a full glass of water to minimize stomach irritation.
- Do NOT crush enteric-coated aspirin.
- Lower doses are recommended for heart attack or stroke prevention.

3. Evaluation: Measuring Treatment Success

- Pain and inflammation are reduced.
- No serious stomach issues or bleeding complications occur.
- Patient understands the importance of proper dosing.

Acetaminophen (Tylenol): A Safe Option for Pain and Fever

Acetaminophen is a widely used pain and fever reliever that does not reduce inflammation like NSAIDs.

It's gentler on the stomach than aspirin but can cause liver damage in high doses.

How Acetaminophen Works (Pharmacodynamics)

- Blocks pain signals in the brain.
- Lowers fever by acting on the hypothalamus (body's temperature control center).

Unlike aspirin, acetaminophen does NOT thin the blood or reduce inflammation.

How Acetaminophen Is Processed (Pharmacokinetics)

- Rapidly absorbed in the stomach and intestines.
- Metabolized by the liver into active and inactive forms.
- Excreted by the kidneys in urine.

High doses can overwhelm the liver, leading to toxicity.

Who Should Use Acetaminophen? (Pharmacotherapeutics)

- Mild to moderate pain relief (headaches, arthritis, toothaches, etc.).
- Fever reduction (preferred option for children).
- Safer alternative for people with ulcers or bleeding risks.

Who Should AVOID Acetaminophen?

- People with liver disease or heavy alcohol use (higher risk of toxicity).
- Patients on high doses of warfarin (possible increased bleeding risk).

Acetaminophen Drug Interactions: What to Watch Out For

Drugs That Can Increase Liver Toxicity:

- Alcohol (even in moderate amounts).
- Seizure medications (phenytoin, carbamazepine).
- Rifampin (used for tuberculosis).

Drugs That May Be Less Effective When Taken with Acetaminophen:

- Loop diuretics (furosemide, bumetanide).
- Zidovudine (used for HIV treatment).

Side Effects of Acetaminophen

Common Side Effects:

- Generally well tolerated in normal doses.

Serious Risks (In High Doses or Overdose):

- Liver failure (can be fatal).
- Severe allergic reactions (rash, blisters, swelling).

Maximum daily dose: 4,000 mg/day for adults (some experts recommend no more than 3,000 mg/day for safety).

Nursing Considerations for Acetaminophen

1. Assessment: Monitoring Patient Safety

- Check total daily intake, including OTC products with hidden acetaminophen.
- Monitor liver function in long-term users.

2. Implementation: Safe Administration

- Use liquid forms for children and patients who have trouble swallowing.
- Do NOT exceed recommended doses.

3. Evaluation: Measuring Treatment Success

- Pain and fever are controlled.
- No signs of liver toxicity occur.
- Patient understands proper dosing and risks.

What Are NSAIDs?

Nonsteroidal anti-inflammatory drugs (NSAIDs) are commonly used to reduce pain, inflammation, and fever. They work by blocking the production of prostaglandins, substances that cause pain and swelling in the body.

Two Types of NSAIDs:

1. Nonselective NSAIDs – Block both COX-1 and COX-2 enzymes.
2. Selective NSAIDs (COX-2 inhibitors) – Only block COX-2, reducing inflammation with less stomach irritation.

Nonselective NSAIDs: Effective But With GI Risks

How They Work (Pharmacodynamics)

Nonselective NSAIDs inhibit both COX-1 and COX-2 enzymes:

- COX-1: Helps protect the stomach lining and regulate blood flow.
- COX-2: Triggers inflammation and pain.

Blocking COX-2 relieves pain, but blocking COX-1 can cause stomach irritation, ulcers, and bleeding.

Common Nonselective NSAIDs

- Ibuprofen (Advil, Motrin)
- Naproxen (Aleve)
- Ketorolac (Toradol)
- Diclofenac (Voltaren)
- Indomethacin
- Meloxicam (Mobic)
- Ketoprofen
- Sulindac

Ibuprofen and naproxen are widely available over-the-counter (OTC), while others require a prescription.

Who Should Use NSAIDs? (Pharmacotherapeutics)

NSAIDs are used for pain relief and inflammation control in:

- Arthritis (osteoarthritis, rheumatoid arthritis)
- Back pain and muscle aches

- Headaches and migraines
- Menstrual cramps
- Tendonitis and bursitis
- Gout
- Mild to moderate post-surgical pain

Who Should AVOID NSAIDs?

- People with stomach ulcers or GI bleeding
- Patients with kidney or liver disease
- People with heart disease or high blood pressure (risk of heart attack and stroke)
- Those taking blood thinners (warfarin, heparin, etc.)

How NSAIDs Are Processed (Pharmacokinetics)

- Absorbed in the stomach and intestines
- Metabolized in the liver
- Excreted by the kidneys

NSAIDs should be taken with food to minimize stomach irritation.

NSAID Drug Interactions: What to Watch Out For

Drugs That Can Cause Serious Side Effects When Combined With NSAIDs:

- Blood thinners (warfarin, heparin) – Increased risk of bleeding.
- Lithium – NSAIDs can increase lithium toxicity.
- ACE inhibitors & beta-blockers – NSAIDs can reduce their effectiveness for high blood pressure.
- Methotrexate – NSAIDs can increase its toxicity.
- Corticosteroids – Higher risk of stomach ulcers.

Common NSAID Side Effects

Mild Side Effects:

- Stomach pain, nausea, and heartburn

- Headache and dizziness
- Fluid retention (swelling in the legs and feet)

Serious Risks (Rare But Dangerous):

- Stomach ulcers and internal bleeding
- High blood pressure and heart failure
- Kidney damage (especially with long-term use)

Long-term NSAID use should be monitored by a doctor to prevent kidney and heart problems.

Nursing Considerations for NSAIDs

1. Assessment: Monitoring Patient Safety

- Check for a history of ulcers, kidney disease, or heart problems.
- Monitor for signs of bleeding (dark stools, stomach pain, easy bruising).
- Assess pain level before and after NSAID use.

2. Implementation: Safe Administration

- Give NSAIDs with food or milk to reduce stomach irritation.
- Have patients drink plenty of water to prevent kidney damage.
- Avoid taking NSAIDs before surgery (increased bleeding risk).

3. Evaluation: Measuring Treatment Success

- Pain and inflammation are reduced.
- No serious stomach, kidney, or heart issues occur.
- Patient understands proper NSAID use and risks.

Selective NSAIDs (COX-2 Inhibitors): Gentler on the Stomach

What Makes COX-2 Inhibitors Different?

- Block only COX-2 (which causes inflammation)
- Preserve COX-1 (which protects the stomach lining)

These NSAIDs cause fewer stomach problems but still pose heart risks.

The Only COX-2 Inhibitor Available Today: Celecoxib (Celebrex)

When Is Celecoxib Used?

- Osteoarthritis and rheumatoid arthritis
- Acute pain and menstrual cramps
- Familial adenomatous polyposis (to prevent colon polyps)

COX-2 Inhibitor Drug Interactions

Drugs That May Cause Serious Interactions With Celecoxib:

- Blood thinners (warfarin, aspirin) – Increased bleeding risk.
- Lithium – Higher risk of toxicity.
- ACE inhibitors & diuretics – Reduced effectiveness for high blood pressure.

Patients with heart disease should avoid COX-2 inhibitors due to increased heart attack risk.

COX-2 Inhibitor Side Effects

Mild Side Effects:

- Upset stomach, nausea, and bloating
- Headache and dizziness

Serious Risks (Rare But Dangerous):

- Heart attack and stroke (higher risk with long-term use)
- High blood pressure and fluid retention

Nursing Considerations for Celecoxib

1. Assessment: Monitoring Patient Safety

- Check for a history of heart disease, high blood pressure, or kidney problems.
- Monitor for swelling, high blood pressure, or chest pain.

2. Implementation: Safe Administration

- Give celecoxib with food to reduce stomach discomfort.
- Do not use in patients with sulfa allergies.
- Monitor kidney function in long-term users.

3. Evaluation: Measuring Treatment Success

- Pain and inflammation are relieved.
- No serious cardiovascular or stomach issues occur.
- Patient understands the risks and benefits of COX-2 inhibitors.

Phenazopyridine: A Urinary Tract Pain Reliever

What Is It Used For?

- Relieves pain, burning, and urgency from urinary tract infections (UTIs).
- Used for short-term symptom relief (does NOT treat infection itself).

How Phenazopyridine Works

- Acts as a local anesthetic in the urinary tract.
- Starts working within 24–48 hours.

It does NOT kill bacteria, so antibiotics are still needed for a UTI.

Important Warnings About Phenazopyridine

- Turns urine red or orange – This is normal but can stain clothes and contact lenses.
- May cause yellowing of skin and eyes if used too long (sign of toxicity).

Nursing Considerations for Phenazopyridine

1. Assessment: Monitoring Patient Safety

- Check for liver or kidney disease (drug is excreted in urine).
- Assess pain levels before and after treatment.

2. Implementation: Safe Administration

- Give with food to reduce nausea.
- Warn patients about urine discoloration.

3. Evaluation: Measuring Treatment Success

- Urinary pain and discomfort are relieved.
- No serious side effects occur.
- Patient understands that an antibiotic is needed to treat the infection itself.

4.3. Opioid Medications: A Guide to Pain Relief and Safety

Opioids are powerful pain relievers derived from the opium plant or synthetic drugs that mimic natural narcotics. They help relieve moderate to severe pain without causing loss of consciousness. Some also suppress coughs and control diarrhea.

Types of Opioid Medications:

1. Opioid Agonists – Strong painkillers that fully activate opioid receptors.
2. Opioid Antagonists – Block opioid effects and reverse overdose.
3. Mixed Opioid Agonist-Antagonists – Relieve pain while reducing risk of addiction and respiratory depression.

1. Opioid Agonists: Powerful Painkillers

How They Work (Pharmacodynamics)

Opioid agonists bind to opioid receptors in the brain and spinal cord. They mimic endorphins, the body's natural pain relievers, to:

- Block pain signals
- Reduce anxiety about pain
- Suppress cough (antitussive effect)

They also slow down the body, causing:

- Respiratory depression (slow breathing)
- Constipation (slows digestion)
- Drowsiness and sedation

Common Opioid Agonists

- Morphine (gold standard for severe pain)
- Fentanyl (strong, fast-acting painkiller)
- Oxycodone (moderate to severe pain, often combined with acetaminophen)
- Hydrocodone (commonly used for pain and cough suppression)
- Methadone (used for pain and opioid addiction treatment)
- Tramadol (milder opioid with lower addiction potential)

Morphine is the standard by which all other painkillers are measured.

How Opioids Are Processed (Pharmacokinetics)

- Absorbed quickly when taken orally, IV, or injected.
- Metabolized in the liver (some break down into active compounds, which can be toxic in kidney failure).
- Excreted by the kidneys and bile.

Meperidine Warning: It breaks down into a toxic metabolite (normeperidine), which can cause seizures if taken for more than 48 hours or in kidney disease.

Who Should Use Opioid Agonists? (Pharmacotherapeutics)

- Severe pain relief (post-surgery, cancer pain, trauma).
- Chronic pain (for patients who don't respond to other medications).
- Cough suppression (certain opioids like codeine).
- Diarrhea control (some opioids slow digestion).
- Heart failure treatment (morphine helps reduce shortness of breath in fluid buildup).

Who Should AVOID Opioids?

- People with lung diseases (asthma, COPD) – Risk of dangerous breathing problems.
- Patients with a history of addiction – High risk of dependence.
- People with head injuries – Opioids can increase brain pressure.

Opioid Drug Interactions: What to Watch Out For

Drugs That Increase the Risk of Side Effects:

- Alcohol & sedatives (benzodiazepines, sleep aids) – Can cause life-threatening respiratory depression.
- Muscle relaxants & antipsychotics – Increased risk of extreme drowsiness.
- MAO inhibitors (certain antidepressants) – Meperidine can cause seizures, coma, and death.

Common Opioid Side Effects

Mild Side Effects:

- Drowsiness and sedation
- Nausea and vomiting
- Constipation
- Itchy skin

Serious Risks (Rare But Dangerous):

- Respiratory depression (slow, shallow breathing) – Can lead to overdose and death.
- Low blood pressure and fainting (orthostatic hypotension).
- Addiction and dependence (higher risk with long-term use).

Nursing Considerations for Opioids

1. Assessment: Monitoring Patient Safety

- Check respiratory rate before giving opioids (hold if below 12 breaths/min).

- Monitor for signs of overdose (slow breathing, blue lips, unresponsiveness).
- Assess pain levels before and after administration.

2. Implementation: Safe Administration

- Give IV opioids slowly to avoid rapid drops in blood pressure.
- Encourage deep breathing and coughing to prevent lung infections.
- Give with food to reduce nausea.
- Provide stool softeners to prevent constipation.

3. Evaluation: Measuring Treatment Success

- Pain relief is achieved.
- Patient has no serious breathing problems.
- No signs of opioid overdose or dependence.

2. Opioid Antagonists: Reversing Overdose & Toxicity

What Do They Do?

Opioid antagonists block opioid receptors, reversing the effects of opioids.

- Used to treat opioid overdose.
- Can also reverse respiratory depression caused by opioid painkillers.
- Works within minutes but may need repeated doses.

Downside: It reverses ALL opioid effects, bringing pain back immediately.

Common Opioid Antagonists

- Naloxone (Narcan) – Fast-acting opioid overdose reversal drug (available as injection or nasal spray).
- Naltrexone – Blocks opioids for long-term addiction treatment (used after detox).

Naloxone works within minutes but wears off quickly, so repeat doses may be needed.

Opioid Antagonist Side Effects

Common Reactions:

- Sudden return of pain
- Nausea, sweating, shaking
- Fast heart rate and high blood pressure

Serious Risks:

- Severe withdrawal symptoms in opioid-dependent patients
- Seizures (rare but possible with high doses)

3. Mixed Opioid Agonist-Antagonists: Safer Pain Control?

How They Work

These drugs activate opioid receptors (for pain relief) while also blocking some effects (to reduce abuse potential).

- Less risk of respiratory depression than full opioids.
- Lower risk of addiction but can still cause dependence.

Not recommended for people already taking opioids – Can trigger withdrawal symptoms.

Common Mixed Opioid Agonist-Antagonists

- Buprenorphine (Suboxone, Subutex) – Used for pain and opioid addiction treatment.
- Butorphanol – Used for migraine pain and labor pain.
- Nalbuphine – Used for moderate pain relief with fewer breathing risks.
- Pentazocine – Combined with naloxone to prevent misuse.

Buprenorphine is a key medication for opioid addiction treatment.

Mixed Opioid Side Effects

Mild Effects:

- Dizziness and sedation
- Nausea and vomiting
- Sweating

Serious Risks:

- Withdrawal symptoms if switching from full opioids.
- Respiratory depression (lower risk than full opioids).

Nursing Considerations for Mixed Opioids

1. Assessment: Monitoring Patient Safety

- Check for prior opioid use (risk of withdrawal symptoms).
- Monitor for respiratory depression and dizziness.

2. Implementation: Safe Administration

- Give IV opioids slowly to reduce dizziness.
- Keep naloxone available in case of overdose.

3. Evaluation: Measuring Treatment Success

- Pain relief is achieved.
- No signs of overdose or respiratory distress.

Opioid Antagonists: Reversing Opioid Effects and Overdose

Opioid antagonists are medications that block the effects of opioids by attaching to opioid receptors without activating them. They work by reversing opioid overdoses, managing opioid dependence, and treating opioid-induced constipation.

Key Opioid Antagonists:

1. Naloxone (Narcan) – Reverses opioid overdose immediately.

2. Naltrexone – Helps prevent opioid relapse in addiction recovery.
3. Methylnaltrexone – Treats opioid-induced constipation without affecting pain relief.

How Opioid Antagonists Work (Pharmacodynamics)

- Block opioid receptors so opioids can't attach.
- Reverse opioid effects like sedation and slow breathing.
- Can bring withdrawal symptoms if opioids are still in the body.

Opioid antagonists DO NOT cause pain relief. Instead, they take away the effects of opioids, including pain relief.

When Are Opioid Antagonists Used? (Pharmacotherapeutics)

1. Opioid Overdose Reversal (Naloxone)

Used in emergency situations to reverse overdose effects like:

- Slow or stopped breathing
- Unresponsiveness
- Pinpoint pupils

Works in minutes but may need repeated doses as opioids last longer than naloxone.

2. Opioid Addiction Treatment (Naltrexone)

- Helps prevent relapse in patients recovering from opioid addiction.
- Only given after detox – If opioids are still in the system, naltrexone can trigger withdrawal symptoms.

3. Opioid-Induced Constipation (Methylnaltrexone)

- Used when laxatives don't work in patients taking long-term opioids.
- Unlike naloxone and naltrexone, methylnaltrexone does NOT affect pain relief.

How Opioid Antagonists Are Processed (Pharmacokinetics)

- Naloxone – Given IV, IM, or subcutaneously, works fast but lasts only 30–90 minutes.
- Naltrexone – Taken orally or as an injectable, lasts 24–48 hours.
- Methylnaltrexone – Taken subcutaneously, works within 30 minutes for constipation relief.

Naloxone is short-acting, so opioid overdose patients may need multiple doses.

Opioid Antagonist Side Effects

Common Side Effects:

- Rapid return of pain
- Nausea and vomiting
- Sweating and chills
- Increased heart rate and blood pressure

Serious Risks (Rare but Important):

- Severe opioid withdrawal symptoms (in dependent patients).
- Respiratory distress if opioid overdose reoccurs after naloxone wears off.

Nursing Considerations for Opioid Antagonists

1. Assessment: Monitoring Patient Safety

- Check for recent opioid use before giving naltrexone (to prevent withdrawal).
- Monitor breathing and oxygen levels before and after naloxone administration.
- Assess hydration status if nausea or diarrhea occurs.

2. Implementation: Safe Administration

- For overdose, give naloxone IM, IV, or nasal spray and repeat as needed.

- For opioid dependence, ensure the patient is fully detoxed before giving naltrexone.
- Monitor blood pressure and heart rate after giving opioid antagonists.

3. Evaluation: Measuring Treatment Success

- Patient's breathing improves after naloxone.
- Patient does not experience severe withdrawal effects.
- Patient understands medication purpose and side effects.

4.4. Anesthetic Drugs: Understanding Their Role in Pain Management

Anesthetic drugs help manage pain by either numbing a specific area or inducing a temporary state of unconsciousness. These drugs are categorized into three main types:

- General Anesthetics – Used for major surgeries, making patients completely unconscious.
- Local Anesthetics – Numb a specific area while the patient remains awake.
- Topical Anesthetics – Applied directly to the skin or mucous membranes for minor procedures.

General Anesthetics: Going Under for Surgery

Inhaled Anesthetics

Common inhalation anesthetics include:

- Desflurane
- Sevoflurane
- Isoflurane
- Nitrous Oxide ("Laughing Gas")

How They Work (Pharmacodynamics)

- Depress the central nervous system (CNS) → Loss of consciousness
- Relax muscles → No movement during surgery
- Reduce pain perception

Serious Risk: Malignant Hyperthermia

- A rare but life-threatening reaction causing high fever and muscle rigidity.
- Dantrolene is the antidote.

Who Should Avoid These Drugs?

- Patients with liver disease
- Patients with a history of malignant hyperthermia
- Pregnant or breastfeeding individuals (use with caution)

After Surgery: Common Side Effects

- Drowsiness & Confusion
- Nausea & Vomiting
- Breathing difficulties (temporary)
- Feeling cold (hypothermia)

IV Anesthetics: Fast-Acting Sedation

Common IV Anesthetics:

- Barbiturates – Thiopental, Methohexital
- Benzodiazepines – Midazolam, Diazepam
- Hypnotics – Propofol, Etomidate
- Opiates – Fentanyl, Sufentanil

How They Work

- Induce sleep quickly
- Shorter duration (used in minor surgeries)

- Often combined with inhaled anesthetics for longer procedures

Propofol Warning: Can cause low blood pressure, slow breathing, and metabolic imbalances (propofol infusion syndrome).

Ketamine: Causes a "dissociative state" – the patient may seem awake but is unaware of surroundings.

Local Anesthetics: Targeted Numbing Without Unconsciousness

Used for procedures like dental work, stitches, and minor surgeries.

Common Local Anesthetics:

- Lidocaine
- Bupivacaine
- Ropivacaine

How They Work

- Block nerve signals in the applied area.
- Prevent the brain from feeling pain at that site.

Potential Risks

- Allergic reactions
- Dizziness & blurred vision
- Irregular heartbeat (rare in high doses)

Nursing Considerations: Keeping Patients Safe

Before Anesthesia

- Check for allergies (especially to local anesthetics)
- Review medical history (heart, lung, or liver disease)
- Ensure the patient has followed pre-surgery fasting guidelines

During Anesthesia

- Monitor breathing & blood pressure closely
- Watch for signs of an allergic reaction

After Anesthesia

- Help the patient wake up safely
- Manage nausea & vomiting
- Encourage deep breathing exercises to prevent lung complications

Topical Anesthetics: How They Work and When to Use Them

Topical anesthetics are pain-relieving medications applied directly to the skin or mucous membranes to numb an area and provide temporary relief from discomfort. These are commonly used for:

- Minor burns and skin irritations
- Itching and rashes
- Numbing before injections
- Sore throat or mouth pain relief
- Numbing before inserting medical tubes (like catheters)

Types of Topical Anesthetics

Common Standalone Topical Anesthetics:

- Benzocaine (often used for mouth and throat pain)
- Lidocaine (used in creams, patches, sprays)
- Dibucaine
- Pramoxine
- Procaine

Combination Products:

- Lidocaine + Prilocaine (commonly used before medical procedures)
- Benzocaine + Menthol (found in lozenges and throat sprays)

Special Forms of Topical Anesthetics:

- Ethyl chloride spray – Freezes the skin for quick numbing

- Menthol-based creams – Creates a cooling effect to reduce discomfort

How Do Topical Anesthetics Work?

Blocking Pain Signals

- These medications prevent nerve signals from reaching the brain, so the treated area feels numb.

Cooling & Counterirritation

- Some anesthetics (like menthol) stimulate cold receptors, creating a cooling sensation that distracts from pain.
- Ethyl chloride spray freezes the skin, numbing the area instantly.

How Are They Used?

Pain & Skin Conditions

- Minor burns and sunburns
- Scrapes, cuts, insect bites
- Poison ivy/oak rash
- Eczema and dermatitis

Before Medical Procedures

- Numbing the skin before injections or minor procedures
- Relieving sore throats (as sprays or lozenges)
- Numbing the eyes before procedures (Tetracaine drops)
- Reducing pain before inserting catheters or tubes

Are There Any Drug Interactions?

Unlike oral or injectable medications, topical anesthetics have very few drug interactions because they are mostly not absorbed into the bloodstream. However:

Caution With Overuse

- Too much topical anesthetic, especially over large areas, can be absorbed into the blood, leading to side effects like dizziness or irregular heartbeat.
- If using multiple numbing products, check labels to avoid overdosing.

Possible Side Effects

Skin Reactions

- Rash, redness, or itching
- Swelling or hives (allergic reaction)
- Skin irritation (from benzyl alcohol)

Too Much Cold Exposure

- Ethyl chloride spray can cause frostbite if left on too long.

Serious Reactions (Rare)

- Severe allergic reactions (difficulty breathing, swelling of the face/throat) → Seek medical help immediately!

Nursing Considerations: Keeping Patients Safe

Before Using the Medication

- Assess the patient's condition – What is the anesthetic needed for?
- Check for allergies – Especially to local anesthetics like lidocaine or benzocaine.
- Review any medical conditions – Patients with heart or liver problems should use caution.

While Using the Medication

- Monitor for skin irritation – Look for rashes, redness, or burning.
- Ensure proper application – Only apply to intact skin (not open wounds, unless directed).
- Watch for overuse – Large applications can lead to toxicity.

After Application

- Check pain relief – Has the anesthetic worked effectively?
- Ensure patient comfort – Avoid contact with eyes unless specifically formulated for eye use.
- Educate the patient – Let them know the numbing effect will wear off after a short period.

Chapter 5: Cardiovascular Medicines

5.1. Cardiovascular Medications: How They Help Your Heart and Circulation

Your cardiovascular system is the lifeline of your body. It includes:

- The heart – pumps blood throughout your body
- Arteries & veins – transport oxygen, nutrients, and hormones
- Capillaries – tiny vessels that allow nutrients and waste exchange
- Lymphatic system – helps remove excess fluid and waste

Because this system plays such a critical role in overall health, any heart or blood vessel problems can lead to serious health conditions like high blood pressure, heart failure, or stroke.

5.2. Inotropic Drugs: Strengthening the Heart's Pumping Power

Inotropic drugs help the heart pump more effectively by influencing the strength of its contractions. Positive inotropic drugs, like cardiac glycosides and phosphodiesterase (PDE) inhibitors, increase the force of the heart's contractions, helping the heart push blood more efficiently through the body.

These drugs are especially important for patients with:

- Heart failure – when the heart is too weak to pump blood effectively
- Atrial fibrillation – an irregular heart rhythm that can cause a fast heartbeat
- Other heart conditions where stronger heart contractions are needed

How Do Inotropic Drugs Help?

- Increase the strength of each heartbeat
- Slow down a fast heart rate (helpful in conditions like atrial fibrillation)
- Prevent fluid buildup (reducing swelling in the legs and lungs)
- Help prevent long-term heart damage (by reducing stress on the heart)

Cardiac Glycosides: A Key Type of Inotropic Drug

Cardiac glycosides, such as digoxin, come from the foxglove plant and are commonly used to treat heart failure and irregular heart rhythms.

How Digoxin Works in the Body

How It's Absorbed & Processed

- Absorption: Digoxin is absorbed differently depending on the form (capsules absorb best, followed by elixirs, then tablets).
- Distribution: Once in the body, digoxin concentrates in the heart, liver, and kidneys but isn't strongly bound to blood proteins.
- Elimination: Mostly excreted by the kidneys, meaning patients with kidney disease may need lower doses.

How It Works in the Heart

- Boosts calcium levels in heart cells, leading to stronger contractions
- Slows the heart rate, giving the heart time to fill with blood before the next beat
- Helps control abnormal rhythms like atrial fibrillation

Who Needs Digoxin?

Digoxin is prescribed for patients with:

- Heart failure – to help the heart beat more effectively

- Atrial fibrillation or atrial flutter – to slow a fast, irregular heartbeat
- Paroxysmal atrial tachycardia – to help manage sudden bursts of fast heart rates

Watch Out for Drug Interactions

Digoxin can interact with many other medications. Some can reduce its effectiveness, while others can increase the risk of toxicity.

Medications That Reduce Digoxin's Effect

- Antacids
- Rifampin
- Certain cholesterol medications (cholestyramine)

Medications That Increase Digoxin Toxicity Risk

- Calcium supplements
- Diuretics (water pills) – can lower potassium levels, making digoxin more toxic
- Beta-blockers & calcium channel blockers – can cause dangerously slow heart rates

Herbal Interactions

- St. John's Wort & ginseng can increase digoxin levels, leading to toxicity.

Recognizing Digoxin Toxicity

Digoxin has a narrow therapeutic range, meaning too much can be dangerous. Doctors carefully monitor blood levels (therapeutic range: 0.5–2 ng/mL).

Signs of Digoxin Toxicity

Early Symptoms:

- Nausea, vomiting, and diarrhea
- Loss of appetite and stomach pain

- Fatigue, dizziness, or confusion

Severe Symptoms:

- Blurred or yellow-tinted vision
- Slow or irregular heartbeat
- Heart block or dangerous arrhythmias

How to Safely Take Digoxin

Before Taking a Dose:

- Check your pulse – If your heart rate is below 60 beats per minute, don't take digoxin and call your doctor.
- Take the same dose at the same time every day to keep levels stable.
- If you miss a dose, don't double up—just take the next dose as scheduled.

Monitoring & Safety Tips:

- Doctors check potassium levels regularly – low potassium increases the risk of digoxin toxicity.
- Stay hydrated – dehydration can make side effects worse.
- Don't take antacids or fiber supplements within 2 hours of digoxin—they can block absorption.

What to Expect with Digoxin Therapy

- It may take a few weeks to feel the full benefits.
- Improved energy levels as your heart pumps more efficiently.
- Report any unusual symptoms (nausea, dizziness, vision changes, or slow heartbeat).

5.3. Antiarrhythmic Drugs: Keeping the Heart in Rhythm

These medications help stabilize the heartbeat by treating irregular heart rhythms (arrhythmias). However, they must be used with caution because they can sometimes cause or worsen the very arrhythmias they aim to treat.

The Risk vs. Benefit Factor

Doctors carefully weigh the benefits of antiarrhythmic therapy against the risks, ensuring that the treatment improves heart function without causing new complications.

The Four Classes of Antiarrhythmic Drugs

Antiarrhythmics are divided into four main classes, based on how they work in the heart:

Class I: Sodium Channel Blockers (subdivided into IA, IB, and IC)

- Control electrical activity in the heart by slowing sodium movement
- Examples: Quinidine, Procainamide, Lidocaine

Class II: Beta-Blockers

- Reduce heart rate and stress on the heart
- Examples: Atenolol, Metoprolol, Propranolol

Class III: Potassium Channel Blockers

- Stabilize heart rhythms by prolonging electrical recovery time
- Examples: Amiodarone, Sotalol

Class IV: Calcium Channel Blockers

- Slow heart rate and electrical conduction
- Examples: Diltiazem, Verapamil

Special Mention: Adenosine

- Adenosine doesn't fit neatly into these classes but is often used to quickly stop an abnormal heart rhythm, such as supraventricular tachycardia (SVT).

Class IA Antiarrhythmics: Slowing the Heart's Electrical Signals

Examples:

- Quinidine
- Procainamide
- Disopyramide

How They Work

These medications alter the heart's electrical signals, slowing the transmission of impulses and helping to prevent rapid or irregular heartbeats.

When Are They Used?

- Premature Ventricular Contractions (PVCs) – early extra beats
- Ventricular Tachycardia – fast heart rhythms from the ventricles
- Atrial Fibrillation/Flutter – irregular or very fast atrial heart rhythms

Watch Out for Drug Interactions!

- Macrolide antibiotics (e.g., erythromycin) can increase the risk of dangerous heart rhythms.
- Verapamil + Disopyramide may worsen heart failure.
- Quinidine + Digoxin can lead to digoxin toxicity (nausea, vision changes, slow heart rate).
- Grapefruit juice can delay the breakdown of quinidine, increasing side effects.

Possible Side Effects

Common:

- Nausea, vomiting, diarrhea
- Bitter taste

- Dizziness

Serious Risks:

- New or worsened arrhythmias
- Low blood pressure
- Heart block (slow or blocked electrical signals)

Class IB Antiarrhythmics: Targeting the Ventricles

Examples:

- Lidocaine (often used in emergency settings)
- Mexiletine

How They Work

These medications help regulate electrical activity in the ventricles, reducing abnormal impulses.

When Are They Used?

- Ventricular Tachycardia
- Ventricular Fibrillation (irregular, chaotic heartbeats that can be fatal)

Watch Out for Drug Interactions!

- Beta-blockers or other antiarrhythmics can increase the risk of a slow heart rate.
- Rifampin can make Mexiletine less effective.
- Theophylline + Mexiletine may lead to dangerous high theophylline levels.

Possible Side Effects

Common:

- Drowsiness, dizziness
- Numbness, tingling

- Nausea

Serious Risks:

- Lidocaine toxicity → confusion, seizures, respiratory distress
- Low blood pressure & slow heart rate

How Nurses & Patients Can Manage Antiarrhythmic Therapy

What Nurses Monitor

- Electrocardiogram (ECG) – to detect changes in heart rhythm
- Heart rate & blood pressure – ensuring the drug isn't slowing the heart too much
- Signs of toxicity – confusion, dizziness, seizures, heart block

How Patients Can Stay Safe

- Take medication exactly as prescribed – Never skip or double a dose
- Avoid grapefruit juice if taking quinidine
- Report symptoms like chest pain, dizziness, fainting, or swelling
- Limit alcohol and caffeine – they can worsen arrhythmias
- Check pulse regularly – If it's too slow (<60 bpm), call your doctor

Long-Term Outlook

- Some patients will only need short-term therapy after a heart event.
- Others may require lifelong medication to keep the heart in rhythm.
- Lifestyle changes (diet, exercise, stress management) can improve heart health and reduce the need for medication.

Class IC Antiarrhythmics Drugs

Class IC antiarrhythmics are powerful medications used to treat serious, stubborn arrhythmias that don't respond well to other treatments.

Commonly Used Class IC Medications

- Flecainide acetate
- Moricizine (a mix of IA, IB, and IC properties)
- Propafenone hydrochloride

How Do Class IC Drugs Work?

These medications slow down the electrical impulses traveling through the heart, helping to control fast and irregular heartbeats.

When Are They Used?

- Life-threatening ventricular arrhythmias
- Certain supraventricular arrhythmias (rapid heart rhythms from above the ventricles)
- Preventing episodes of PSVT (Paroxysmal Supraventricular Tachycardia) in patients without structural heart disease

Watch Out for Drug Interactions

- Flecainide & Propafenone + Digoxin → Increases risk of digoxin toxicity
- Quinidine + Propafenone → May lead to dangerously high levels of Propafenone
- Cimetidine + Moricizine → Raises toxicity risk
- Propafenone + Warfarin → Increases blood-thinning effects
- Theophylline + Moricizine → Lowers theophylline levels, reducing its effectiveness

Possible Side Effects of Class IC Drugs

Heart-Related Risks

- New or worsening arrhythmias

- Palpitations & chest pain
- Shortness of breath
- Heart failure

Other Risks

- Dizziness, nausea, vomiting
- Stomach pain, heartburn
- Propafenone may cause bronchospasms (wheezing & difficulty breathing)

Who Should NOT Take Class IC Drugs?

- Patients with structural heart disease (higher risk of death)
- People with recent heart attacks

How Nurses & Patients Can Manage Class IC Therapy

What Nurses Monitor

- Heart rhythm (ECG monitoring) – Checking for any dangerous changes
- Blood pressure & pulse – Ensuring they don't drop too low
- Signs of toxicity – Unusual tiredness, confusion, vision changes
- Electrolyte levels – Low potassium & magnesium can increase risks

Class II Antiarrhythmics: The Beta-Blockers

These slow down the heart rate and reduce the workload on the heart.

Commonly Used Class II Medications

- Propranolol
- Esmolol (IV use only)
- Acebutolol (not commonly used)

How Do Class II Drugs Work?

They block beta receptors, which slows down the electrical signals in the heart, reducing:

- Automaticity (how fast the heart fires electrical signals)
- The force of heart contractions
- The amount of oxygen the heart needs

When Are They Used?

- Atrial fibrillation/flutter (to slow the heart rate)
- Paroxysmal Atrial Tachycardia (PAT)
- Arrhythmias from too much adrenaline (e.g., stress-induced arrhythmias)

Watch Out for Drug Interactions

- Beta-blockers + Other Blood Pressure Medications → Can cause low blood pressure
- Beta-blockers + NSAIDs → May reduce effectiveness
- Propranolol + Verapamil → Can cause dangerous slowing of the heart
- Esmolol + Digoxin → May increase digoxin toxicity

Possible Side Effects of Class II Drugs

Heart-Related Risks

- Slow heart rate (bradycardia)
- Low blood pressure
- Heart failure (in some cases)

Other Risks

- Dizziness, fatigue
- Bronchospasm (wheezing, difficulty breathing) – Especially in asthma patients
- Nausea, diarrhea

Who Should NOT Take Class II Drugs?

- People with asthma (due to bronchospasm risk)
- Patients with severe heart failure

How Nurses & Patients Can Manage Class II Therapy

What Nurses Monitor

- Heart rate & blood pressure – If too low, the drug may need to be stopped
- Breathing difficulties – Watching for signs of wheezing
- Signs of heart failure – Swelling, weight gain, extreme fatigue

What Patients Should Do

- Take at the same time daily
- Do NOT stop suddenly (can cause dangerous heart problems)
- Check pulse regularly (notify doctor if below 60 bpm)
- Avoid excessive caffeine & alcohol

Class IV Antiarrhythmics: Calcium Channel Blockers

Class IV antiarrhythmic drugs are calcium channel blockers that help manage certain types of fast heart rhythms. The two most commonly used medications in this class are:

- Verapamil
- Diltiazem

How Do They Work?

These drugs slow down the movement of calcium into the heart and blood vessel walls, which:

- Reduces heart rate
- Lowers blood pressure

- Decreases oxygen demand on the heart
- Helps restore a normal rhythm

When Are They Used?

- Supraventricular arrhythmias – Rapid heart rhythms originating above the ventricles
- Angina – Chest pain caused by reduced blood flow to the heart
- Hypertension – High blood pressure
- Atrial fibrillation/flutter – To help slow the heart rate

Drug Interactions to Watch For

- Verapamil + Beta Blockers → Can slow the heart rate too much
- Diltiazem + Digoxin → May increase digoxin levels (risk of toxicity)
- Calcium Channel Blockers + Anesthetics → Can enhance the effects of anesthesia
- Diltiazem + Cyclosporine → Increases risk of toxicity
- Verapamil + Alcohol → Enhances alcohol's effects
- Grapefruit Juice + Verapamil → May increase drug levels and cause toxicity

Possible Side Effects

Mild Effects

- Dizziness
- Headache
- Low blood pressure
- Constipation
- Nausea
- Rash

Serious Risks

- Heart failure

- Slow heart rate (bradycardia)
- Heart block (AV block)
- Severe low blood pressure
- Fluid buildup in the lungs (pulmonary edema)

Who Should Avoid Class IV Drugs?

- People with severe heart failure
- Patients with low blood pressure
- Those with certain types of heart block

Managing Class IV Therapy: What Nurses & Patients Should Know

What Nurses Monitor

- Heart rhythm & ECG – Watching for dangerous rhythm changes
- Blood pressure – Ensuring it doesn't drop too low
- Signs of fluid retention – Swelling, shortness of breath
- Kidney & liver function – Monitoring metabolism & excretion

What Patients Should Do

- Take medication at the same time every day
- Avoid grapefruit juice
- Monitor for dizziness or fatigue
- Check with a doctor before stopping the drug

Adenosine: A Special Antiarrhythmic Drug

Adenosine is a rapid-acting injectable drug used for emergency treatment of Paroxysmal Supraventricular Tachycardia (PSVT).

How Does It Work?

- Slows conduction through the AV node
- Interrupts abnormal fast rhythms

- Temporarily "resets" the heart's electrical activity

When Is It Used?

- PSVT (Paroxysmal Supraventricular Tachycardia)
- Wolff-Parkinson-White (WPW) Syndrome (Abnormal heart pathways causing fast rhythms)

Works within seconds! But the effects only last a few minutes.

Drug Interactions with Adenosine

- Methylxanthines (Caffeine, Theophylline) → Reduce effectiveness
- Dipyridamole (Blood thinner) → Enhances effects (Smaller dose needed)
- Carbamazepine (Seizure drug) → Increases risk of heart block

Possible Side Effects

- Flushing (warm sensation in face/neck)
- Shortness of breath
- Dizziness
- Chest pain (brief but can feel scary!)
- Lightheadedness or fainting

These symptoms usually last less than 1 minute!

Managing Adenosine Therapy

What Nurses Monitor

- Heart rhythm (ECG monitoring) – Ensuring the heart returns to normal
- Blood pressure & pulse – Watching for sudden drops
- Breathing difficulties – Some patients may feel short of breath

What Patients Should Expect

- A brief "pause" in the heartbeat (can feel like a mild "shock")

- A warm flush or chest discomfort for a few seconds
- Heart rhythm should return to normal quickly

Adenosine is fast-acting, but close monitoring is required!

5.4. Antianginal drugs

Angina, or chest pain, is a sign that the heart isn't getting enough oxygen. While pain relief is crucial, antianginal drugs don't just mask the pain—they actually help the heart work more efficiently by:

- Reducing how much oxygen the heart needs
- Increasing oxygen supply to the heart
- Improving blood flow

Types of Antianginal Drugs

There are three main classes of antianginal medications:

1. Nitrates – Used immediately to relieve chest pain.
2. Beta Blockers – Prevent angina in the long run.
3. Calcium Channel Blockers – Used if other drugs don't fully control angina.

Nitrates: The First Line of Defense

Nitrates are the go-to drugs for stopping an angina attack fast. They help relax and widen blood vessels, improving blood flow and reducing the heart's workload.

Common Nitrates

- Nitroglycerin (most commonly used)
- Isosorbide dinitrate
- Isosorbide mononitrate
- Amyl nitrite

How Do Nitrates Work?

- Relax blood vessels (vasodilation) → Less strain on the heart

- Reduce blood returning to the heart (preload) → Eases workload
- Lower resistance in arteries (afterload) → Allows blood to flow more easily

Result: Less oxygen demand, less chest pain!

How Nitrates Are Taken

Fast relief options (for sudden angina attacks):

- Sublingual tablets (under the tongue)
- Lingual sprays (sprayed under the tongue)
- Buccal tablets (placed inside the cheek)
- Amyl nitrite inhalation (rarely used)

Long-acting options (to prevent angina):

- Oral capsules
- Patches (applied to the skin)
- Ointments (rubbed on the skin)

Emergency option:

- IV nitroglycerin (used in hospitals for severe cases)

Drug Interactions to Watch For

Severe low blood pressure (hypotension) risk with:

- Alcohol
- Sildenafil (Viagra) or other ED drugs (must wait 24 hours before taking nitrates!)
- Calcium channel blockers (can cause dizzy spells or fainting)

Side Effects of Nitrates

Common Effects

- Headaches (most common – goes away with time)
- Dizziness or fainting
- Flushing (red, warm skin)

- Increased heart rate

Serious Effects

- Severe drop in blood pressure
- Fainting when standing up (orthostatic hypotension)
- Heart palpitations

Tip: Sit or lie down when taking your first nitrate dose to avoid dizziness.

How to Use Nitrates Safely

For fast relief (sublingual nitroglycerin)

- Place 1 tablet under the tongue and let it dissolve.
- If pain doesn't go away in 5 minutes, take another dose.
- You can take up to 3 doses (every 5 minutes).

For patches/ointments

- Rotate where you place the patch (to avoid skin irritation).
- Remove patches before sleep (prevents "tolerance" to nitrates).
- Remove before defibrillation! (Patches have metal and can cause burns.)

Beta Blockers: Long-Term Angina Prevention

Beta blockers don't provide immediate relief, but they prevent angina by reducing:

- Heart rate (so the heart works less)
- Blood pressure
- The force of heart contractions

Common Beta Blockers for Angina

- Atenolol
- Metoprolol
- Propranolol
- Carvedilol

- Nadolol

Beta Blocker Interactions & Side Effects

- NSAIDs (like ibuprofen) → Can reduce the effect of beta blockers
- Diabetes medications → Beta blockers can hide symptoms of low blood sugar
- Other heart medications → May slow the heart too much
- DO NOT STOP SUDDENLY – Stopping abruptly can cause dangerous heart problems!

Calcium Channel Blockers: An Alternative Option

If nitrates and beta blockers aren't enough, calcium channel blockers may be added. These drugs relax blood vessels and reduce heart workload.

Common Calcium Channel Blockers for Angina

- Amlodipine
- Diltiazem
- Nifedipine
- Verapamil

How Calcium Channel Blockers Work

- Relax & widen blood vessels → More oxygen to the heart
- Lower blood pressure → Heart doesn't have to work as hard
- Slow heart rate (some types) → Less oxygen demand

Not for immediate relief of chest pain!

Drug Interactions & Side Effects

- Grapefruit juice → Can increase the risk of side effects
- Calcium supplements → Can reduce effectiveness
- Beta blockers → May cause slow heart rate or heart block

Common Side Effects

- Swelling in legs (fluid retention)
- Dizziness or lightheadedness
- Constipation (with verapamil)

Serious Effects

- Severe low blood pressure
- Worsening heart failure
- Abnormal heart rhythms

5.5. Antihypertensive drugs

High blood pressure (hypertension) is a silent but serious condition. Left untreated, it can lead to heart disease, stroke, kidney damage, and other complications. Luckily, a variety of antihypertensive medications can help keep blood pressure under control.

Types of Antihypertensive Drugs

Doctors may prescribe one or more of the following main drug classes to manage high blood pressure:

1. Diuretics – Often the first-line treatment.
2. Angiotensin-Converting Enzyme (ACE) Inhibitors – Helps relax blood vessels.
3. Angiotensin II Receptor Blockers (ARBs) – Works similarly to ACE inhibitors.
4. Beta Blockers – Slows heart rate and reduces workload on the heart.
5. Calcium Channel Blockers – Prevents blood vessels from narrowing.

If these aren't effective alone, other additional options include:

- Sympatholytic drugs (affect the nervous system)
- Direct vasodilators (help blood vessels relax)
- Selective aldosterone-receptor antagonists (reduce sodium and water retention)

ACE Inhibitors: Keeping Blood Pressure in Check

ACE inhibitors are among the most commonly prescribed antihypertensives. They lower blood pressure by blocking the production of angiotensin II, a hormone that makes blood vessels tighten.

Common ACE Inhibitors

- Captopril
- Enalapril
- Lisinopril
- Ramipril
- Quinapril
- Benazepril
- Fosinopril

How ACE Inhibitors Work

- Blocks angiotensin II production → Blood vessels relax → Lower blood pressure
- Reduces sodium & water retention → Less fluid → Less strain on the heart
- Increases blood flow → Reduces the risk of heart damage

Result: Lower blood pressure & better heart function!

ACE Inhibitor Drug Interactions

Potential risks with:

- Diuretics & other antihypertensives → May drop blood pressure too much
- NSAIDs (ibuprofen, naproxen) → May reduce ACE inhibitor effectiveness
- Potassium supplements or potassium-sparing diuretics → Risk of high potassium levels

- Lithium → ACE inhibitors can increase lithium levels (risk of toxicity!)

Side Effects of ACE Inhibitors

Common Effects

- Persistent dry cough
- Dizziness or lightheadedness
- Fatigue
- Mild swelling in hands/feet

Serious Effects (Less Common)

- Severe drop in blood pressure (hypotension)
- High potassium levels (hyperkalemia)
- Kidney problems
- Angioedema (swelling of the lips, face, or throat – seek emergency care!)

Pregnant women should AVOID ACE inhibitors! They can harm fetal circulation.

How to Take ACE Inhibitors Safely

Take on an empty stomach (30 minutes before or 1-2 hours after meals).

- Check your blood pressure regularly.
- Drink plenty of fluids (but not too much potassium!).
- Avoid sudden movements (stand up slowly to prevent dizziness).
- Don't stop suddenly – stopping abruptly can cause a dangerous rise in blood pressure!

Angiotensin II Receptor Blockers (ARBs): An Alternative to ACE Inhibitors

If ACE inhibitors cause side effects (like a chronic cough), ARBs are a great alternative. They work similarly but don't block ACE directly, which means fewer side effects.

Common ARBs

- Losartan
- Valsartan
- Irbesartan
- Olmesartan
- Telmisartan

How ARBs Work

- Block angiotensin II receptors → Prevents blood vessels from tightening
- Lowers blood pressure (similar to ACE inhibitors)
- Reduces strain on the heart

Key Difference: ARBs don't cause the dry cough that ACE inhibitors do.

ARB Drug Interactions

- NSAIDs → May reduce effectiveness.
- Diuretics or beta blockers → May drop blood pressure too much.
- Potassium supplements → Can cause high potassium levels.

Side Effects of ARBs

Common Effects

- Dizziness
- Fatigue
- Mild swelling in hands/feet

Serious Effects

- Low blood pressure
- Kidney problems
- High potassium levels

Like ACE inhibitors, ARBs should NOT be taken during pregnancy!

Beta Blockers: Slowing Things Down

Beta blockers slow the heart rate and reduce how hard the heart pumps, making them useful for both hypertension & heart disease.

Common Beta Blockers

- Atenolol
- Metoprolol
- Propranolol
- Nadolol

How Beta Blockers Work

- Slow the heart rate → Heart needs less oxygen
- Reduce blood pressure → Less strain on blood vessels
- Prevent chest pain & heart attacks

Not for everyone! Beta blockers are NOT recommended for people with asthma or severe lung disease because they can make breathing more difficult.

Beta Blocker Drug Interactions

- Diabetes medications → May hide symptoms of low blood sugar.
- Other heart medications → May slow the heart too much.
- NSAIDs → Can reduce effectiveness.

Side Effects of Beta Blockers

Common Effects

- Fatigue

- Cold hands & feet
- Dizziness
- Mild weight gain

Serious Effects

- Very slow heart rate (bradycardia)
- Shortness of breath
- Worsening heart failure

DO NOT STOP SUDDENLY! Stopping a beta blocker suddenly can cause a dangerous rebound in blood pressure & heart rate.

Calcium Channel Blockers: Another Option for Hypertension

Calcium channel blockers prevent blood vessels from tightening, making them another good option for lowering blood pressure.

Common Calcium Channel Blockers

- Amlodipine
- Diltiazem
- Nifedipine
- Verapamil

How Calcium Channel Blockers Work

- Relax & widen blood vessels → More oxygen to the heart
- Lower blood pressure → Heart doesn't have to work as hard
- Some slow the heart rate (diltiazem, verapamil)

Not for immediate relief of high blood pressure!

Side Effects of Calcium Channel Blockers

Common Effects

- Swelling in legs (fluid retention)
- Dizziness
- Constipation (with verapamil)

Serious Effects

- Severe low blood pressure
- Worsening heart failure
- Abnormal heart rhythms

Calcium channel blockers

Managing high blood pressure (hypertension) is crucial for heart health, stroke prevention, and overall well-being. There are several categories of medications that work in different ways to lower blood pressure. This guide breaks them down in simple terms to help you understand their role, how they work, and what to watch for.

Helping Blood Flow Freely

Calcium channel blockers (CCBs) are widely used to treat high blood pressure. They also help prevent chest pain (angina) and control abnormal heart rhythms (arrhythmias).

Common Calcium Channel Blockers

- Amlodipine
- Diltiazem
- Felodipine
- Nifedipine
- Verapamil

How They Work

- Relax & widen blood vessels → Lower blood pressure
- Reduce the force of heart contractions → Less strain on the heart
- Some (diltiazem & verapamil) slow heart rate → Reduce oxygen demand

Result: Improved circulation, reduced blood pressure, and prevention of chest pain.

Drug Interactions

- Medications & substances that may interfere with calcium channel blockers:
- Calcium supplements & vitamin D → May reduce drug effectiveness
- Digoxin & diltiazem/verapamil → Increases the risk of digoxin toxicity
- Grapefruit juice → May increase drug levels (avoid it!)

Possible Side Effects

Common Effects

- Dizziness & headaches
- Swelling in legs (fluid retention)
- Flushing & palpitations
- Mild nausea

Serious Effects (Less Common)

- Severe low blood pressure
- Worsening heart failure
- Abnormal heart rhythms (bradycardia, AV block)

If you feel lightheaded, have severe swelling, or experience chest pain, contact your doctor!

How to Take Calcium Channel Blockers Safely

- Take with or without food (except amlodipine, which should not be taken with high-fat meals).
- Do not crush or chew extended-release tablets.
- Limit sodium & fluid intake if swelling occurs.
- Stand up slowly to avoid dizziness.
- Check your blood pressure & heart rate regularly.

Diuretics: The "Water Pills"

Diuretics help the body get rid of excess fluid by increasing urine output. This reduces blood volume, which helps lower blood pressure.

Types of Diuretics

- Thiazide diuretics (first-line treatment for hypertension)
- Loop diuretics (used for severe fluid retention)
- Potassium-sparing diuretics (help balance potassium levels)

How They Work

- Flush out extra fluid & salt → Lower blood volume → Lower blood pressure
- Reduce swelling (edema) → Helpful for heart failure

Important Note: Diuretics can cause dehydration & potassium imbalances.

Drug Interactions

- NSAIDs → May reduce diuretic effectiveness
- ACE inhibitors & potassium-sparing diuretics → Risk of high potassium levels
- Lithium → Diuretics can raise lithium levels (risk of toxicity)

Possible Side Effects

Common Effects

- Frequent urination
- Mild dehydration
- Muscle cramps (low potassium)
- Dizziness or weakness

Serious Effects (Less Common)

- Severe dehydration
- Extreme potassium imbalances
- Irregular heartbeats

Drink plenty of water & get blood tests to monitor electrolytes!

Sympatholytic Drugs: Calming the Nervous System

Sympatholytic drugs lower blood pressure by blocking the effects of stress hormones (like adrenaline).

Types of Sympatholytic Drugs

- Alpha-blockers (e.g., doxazosin, prazosin, terazosin) – Relaxes blood vessels.
- Beta-blockers (e.g., propranolol, metoprolol) – Slows heart rate & lowers blood pressure.
- Mixed alpha- & beta-blockers (labetalol, carvedilol) – Works on both blood vessels & heart.

How They Work

- Block stress hormones → Lowers heart rate & blood pressure
- Relax blood vessels → Easier blood flow
- Reduce strain on the heart

Caution: These drugs may cause dizziness, fatigue, and sudden drops in blood pressure.

Drug Interactions

- Beta-blockers & calcium channel blockers → May slow heart rate too much
- Clonidine & beta-blockers → Stopping suddenly can cause a dangerous rise in blood pressure
- Carvedilol & diabetes medications → May increase the risk of low blood sugar

Possible Side Effects

Common Effects

- Drowsiness & fatigue
- Dizziness (especially when standing up too quickly)
- Mild swelling in the feet

Serious Effects (Less Common)

- Severe drop in blood pressure
- Slow heart rate (bradycardia)
- Shortness of breath (especially in asthma patients)

Take at bedtime to reduce dizziness & avoid sudden movements!

Direct Vasodilators: Expanding Blood Vessels

These drugs work by directly relaxing blood vessels, helping reduce resistance and lower blood pressure.

Common Direct Vasodilators

- Hydralazine
- Minoxidil
- Nitroprusside (used in emergencies)

How They Work

- Relax the smooth muscle in blood vessels → Lower blood pressure
- Improve circulation → Reduce strain on the heart

Typically used for severe or resistant hypertension.

Drug Interactions

- Other blood pressure meds → May cause excessive low blood pressure
- Diuretics → Helps prevent fluid buildup from vasodilators

Possible Side Effects

Common Effects

- Headache & flushing
- Rapid heartbeat (palpitations)
- Water retention & swelling

Serious Effects (Less Common)

- Chest pain
- Severe fluid retention
- Excessive hair growth (minoxidil side effect)

Regular check-ups are needed to monitor side effects!

Managing Blood Pressure with Special Medications

Managing blood pressure isn't just about popping a pill—it's about making informed choices, monitoring for side effects, and ensuring medications work effectively. This guide will help break down two types of medications:

1. Nitroprusside & Light-Sensitive IV Medications
2. Selective Aldosterone-Receptor Antagonists (Eplerenone)

Nitroprusside: A High-Power IV Drug for Blood Pressure Emergencies

Nitroprusside is a potent medication used to quickly lower dangerously high blood pressure (hypertensive crisis). Since it works fast, it requires careful monitoring.

How It Works

- Relaxes blood vessels → Lowers blood pressure immediately
- Reduces stress on the heart → Improves blood flow
- Short-acting → Effects wear off quickly when stopped

Special Handling & Administration

- Protect it from light! Nitroprusside is highly sensitive to light.
- Wrap IV bags in foil to prevent breakdown.
- Check the color – it should have a light brown tint. If it looks blue, green, or dark brown, discard it!
- Use an Infusion Pump for Precise Control!
- Given through a dedicated IV line (no mixing with other meds).

- Start slow & adjust based on blood pressure readings.
- Monitor Blood Pressure Closely!
- Check BP every 5 minutes at the start, then every 15 minutes during infusion.
- If BP drops too low, stop the infusion immediately—it wears off quickly due to its short half-life.
- Watch for Cyanide Toxicity!
- If symptoms occur (nausea, confusion, fast heart rate, seizures), stop the drug and notify the doctor immediately.

Supporting a Healthy Blood Pressure Lifestyle

Medication alone isn't enough! Help boost your results with:

- Low-sodium diet (less processed foods, more fresh options)
- Exercise (walking, swimming, yoga—whatever you enjoy!)
- Stress reduction (deep breathing, meditation, fun hobbies)

If using a nitroprusside patch:

- Apply a new patch in a different location each week.
- Remove before defibrillation

Eplerenone: The Selective Aldosterone-Receptor Antagonist

Eplerenone is a special blood pressure medication that helps regulate fluid balance and blood pressure by blocking aldosterone (a hormone that makes the body hold onto salt and water).

How It Works

- Blocks aldosterone → Less fluid retention, lower blood pressure
- Reduces strain on the heart → Helpful for certain heart conditions

Main Concern: High potassium levels (hyperkalemia)!

Drug Interactions & What to Avoid

Avoid these while on eplerenone:

- Potassium supplements or potassium-rich salt substitutes (risk of dangerously high potassium).
- CYP3A4 inhibitors like erythromycin, saquinavir, verapamil, and fluconazole (can raise drug levels too high).

Watch for These Side Effects

Common Reactions:

- Mild fatigue
- Upset stomach or diarrhea
- Tickling cough

Serious Reactions (Call Your Doctor!):

- Irregular heartbeat (possible high potassium levels)
- Unusual swelling or rapid weight gain
- Severe dizziness or confusion

How to Take It Safely

- Take with food or at bedtime to reduce stomach discomfort.
- Stand up slowly to avoid dizziness from low blood pressure.
- Check blood potassium levels regularly to ensure safety.

If you feel extremely weak, confused, or notice irregular heartbeats—seek medical attention ASAP!

5.6. Cholesterol-Lowering Medications

Keeping your cholesterol levels in check is key to heart health and reducing the risk of coronary artery disease (CAD). Antilipemic drugs help lower bad cholesterol (LDL) and triglycerides while boosting good cholesterol (HDL). But they work best when combined with lifestyle changes like a healthy diet, exercise, and weight management.

Types of Cholesterol-Lowering Medications

These medications fall into five major categories, each working in a unique way:

1. Bile-sequestering drugs – Bind to bile acids to remove excess cholesterol.
2. Fibric acid derivatives – Target triglycerides and boost good cholesterol.
3. Statins (HMG-CoA reductase inhibitors) – Block cholesterol production in the liver.
4. Nicotinic acid (Niacin) – Helps increase HDL and lower triglycerides.
5. Cholesterol absorption inhibitors – Reduce cholesterol absorption in the intestines.

1. Bile-Sequestering Drugs: Removing Cholesterol from the Body

These medications, including cholestyramine, colesevelam, and colestipol, don't get absorbed into the bloodstream. Instead, they stay in the intestines, where they bind to bile acids and prevent cholesterol from being reabsorbed.

How They Work

- Bind to bile acids → Prevents the body from reusing them.
- Forces the liver to make more bile acids → Uses up cholesterol in the process.
- Lowers LDL cholesterol → Reduces the risk of heart disease.

Important to Know: These drugs aren't absorbed, so they have fewer systemic side effects but can interfere with fat digestion and vitamin absorption.

Common Drug Interactions

- Can block the absorption of other medications like digoxin, propranolol, and diuretics – Take them 1 hour before or 4-6 hours after bile-sequestering drugs.

- Reduces absorption of fat-soluble vitamins (A, D, E, K) – Long-term use may require supplements.
- Can increase bleeding risk if vitamin K levels drop.

Possible Side Effects

Short-term (Mild):

- Bloating
- Gas
- Nausea

Long-term (More Serious):

- Constipation
- Vitamin deficiencies
- Gallbladder issues

How to Take It Safely

- Mix powdered forms with at least 4–6 oz of liquid (never take dry powder alone!).
- Use a non-carbonated beverage (carbonation can cause foaming).
- If constipation occurs, increase fiber, fluids, or use a stool softener.
- Monitor cholesterol levels every 4–6 weeks to track progress.

2. Fibric Acid Derivatives: Targeting Triglycerides

These drugs—fenofibrate and gemfibrozil—focus on lowering triglycerides while offering a modest LDL reduction and increasing HDL ("good" cholesterol).

How They Work

- Reduce cholesterol production early in its formation.
- Help the body get rid of excess cholesterol through bile.

- Break down triglycerides more efficiently.
- Boost HDL cholesterol, improving overall lipid balance.

Common Drug Interactions

- May interfere with blood thinners like warfarin, increasing the risk of bleeding.
- Shouldn't be combined with statins due to the risk of muscle damage (myopathy or rhabdomyolysis).

Possible Side Effects

- GI issues – Nausea, diarrhea, stomach pain.
- Liver effects – Elevated liver enzymes (needs monitoring).
- Muscle pain or weakness – Report immediately if this occurs.

How to Take It Safely

- Take fenofibrate with food to improve absorption.
- Take gemfibrozil 30 minutes before meals.
- Monitor liver function tests and muscle pain symptoms regularly.
- Stick to a triglyceride-lowering diet for best results.

3. Statins: The Gold Standard for Cholesterol Control

Also called HMG-CoA reductase inhibitors, statins block cholesterol production in the liver. These include:

- Atorvastatin
- Simvastatin
- Rosuvastatin
- Pravastatin
- Fluvastatin

How They Work

- Reduce LDL ("bad" cholesterol) by up to 60%.

- Lower triglycerides modestly.
- Increase HDL ("good" cholesterol).
- Reduce the risk of heart attacks and strokes.

Common Drug Interactions

- Can interact with grapefruit juice – Avoid grapefruit while on statins.
- Don't take with niacin or fibric acid drugs – Can increase muscle damage risk.
- May increase blood sugar levels – Monitor if you have diabetes.

Possible Side Effects

- Muscle pain or weakness – Could signal rhabdomyolysis (a serious muscle breakdown condition).
- Liver enzyme changes – Regular liver function tests recommended.
- GI discomfort – Mild nausea, bloating, or diarrhea.

How to Take It Safely

- Take statins in the evening (cholesterol production is highest at night).
- Stick to a heart-healthy diet for the best effects.
- Monitor liver function and muscle symptoms regularly.

4. Cholesterol Absorption Inhibitors: Stopping Absorption in the Gut

Ezetimibe (Zetia) is the primary drug in this class.

How It Works

- Blocks cholesterol absorption in the intestines.
- Reduces LDL by about 18%.
- Used alone or with statins for extra cholesterol-lowering power.

Possible Side Effects

- Mild stomach upset.
- Liver enzyme changes (when combined with statins).

How to Take It Safely

Take at the same time each day, with or without food.

Regular cholesterol monitoring ensures effectiveness.

Nicotinic Acid & Cholesterol Absorption Inhibitors

Keeping your cholesterol and triglycerides in check is crucial for maintaining heart health and preventing coronary artery disease (CAD). Let's dive into how nicotinic acid (niacin) and cholesterol absorption inhibitors work to keep your lipid levels balanced.

Nicotinic Acid (Niacin): A Vitamin with a Big Impact

Also known as niacin, nicotinic acid is a water-soluble B vitamin that helps to:

- Lower triglycerides (bad fats in the blood).
- Reduce apolipoprotein B-100 (a protein linked to LDL cholesterol).
- Boost HDL (good cholesterol) to help remove bad cholesterol from the body.

How It Works

While the exact mechanism isn't fully understood, niacin may work by:

- Blocking the liver from making too many lipoproteins (which carry cholesterol in the blood).
- Encouraging fat breakdown and removal.
- Increasing the excretion of sterols (a type of fat).

Niacin is available in both immediate-release and extended-release forms, with the latter designed to reduce side effects like flushing.

Drug Interactions

- Combining niacin with statins (HMG-CoA inhibitors) may increase the risk of muscle damage (myopathy or rhabdomyolysis).
- Bile acid sequestrants (like cholestyramine) can reduce niacin's effectiveness – take them several hours apart.
- Kava may increase the risk of liver damage when taken with niacin.

Possible Side Effects

- Flushing and warmth of the face and neck (common with immediate-release niacin).
- Liver toxicity (higher risk with extended-release forms).
- Nausea, vomiting, diarrhea, and stomach pain.

How to Take Niacin Safely

- Take with food to minimize stomach upset.
- Aspirin (taken 30 minutes before niacin) can help reduce flushing.
- Avoid alcohol, spicy foods, and hot drinks before taking niacin to minimize flushing.
- Monitor liver function regularly, as niacin can increase liver enzymes.

Cholesterol Absorption Inhibitors: Blocking the Bad Stuff

A newer class of cholesterol-lowering drugs, cholesterol absorption inhibitors work by preventing cholesterol from being absorbed in the intestines.

- Ezetimibe (Zetia) is the only drug in this class.

How It Works

- Prevents cholesterol absorption in the small intestine.

- Reduces LDL ("bad cholesterol").
- Boosts cholesterol clearance from the liver.
- Can be used alone or with a statin for extra cholesterol-lowering effects.

Drug Interactions

- Cholestyramine and other bile acid sequestrants can decrease ezetimibe's effectiveness – take them several hours apart.
- Fenofibrate and gemfibrozil may increase ezetimibe levels, leading to a higher risk of side effects.
- When combined with statins, ezetimibe may increase the risk of muscle pain and liver enzyme elevation.

Possible Side Effects

- Fatigue, stomach pain, and diarrhea.
- Sinus infections and pharyngitis (sore throat).
- Muscle pain, especially when combined with statins.
- Upper respiratory infections (cold-like symptoms).

How to Take Ezetimibe Safely

- Take at the same time each day, with or without food.
- If using with a statin, monitor for muscle pain.
- Regular cholesterol and liver enzyme tests ensure safety and effectiveness.

Chapter 6: Respiratory Medicines

6.1. Medications for the Respiratory System

The respiratory system plays a crucial role in our daily lives, helping us breathe by taking in oxygen and expelling carbon dioxide. It stretches from the nose and airways down to the tiny pulmonary capillaries in the lungs, ensuring our body gets the oxygen it needs.

When breathing becomes difficult due to conditions like asthma, chronic obstructive pulmonary disease (COPD), or congestion from a cold, medications can help open airways, reduce inflammation, and ease symptoms. These drugs come in different forms, such as inhalers, pills, and syrups, to suit various needs.

Common types of respiratory medications include:

- Beta$_2$-adrenergic agonists – Help relax and widen the airways, making breathing easier (e.g., albuterol, salmeterol).
- Anticholinergics – Reduce mucus production and help open the airways, often used in COPD (e.g., ipratropium, tiotropium).
- Corticosteroids – Reduce airway inflammation to prevent or control asthma and other lung conditions (e.g., prednisone, fluticasone).
- Leukotriene modifiers – Block substances that trigger inflammation and constriction in the lungs (e.g., montelukast).
- Mast cell stabilizers – Help prevent allergic reactions that cause airway tightening (e.g., cromolyn sodium).
- Methylxanthines – Work as bronchodilators to help keep airways open for easier breathing (e.g., theophylline).
- Expectorants – Loosen mucus, making it easier to clear from the airways (e.g., guaifenesin).

- Antitussives – Suppress coughing when it becomes excessive or painful (e.g., dextromethorphan, codeine).
- Decongestants – Reduce swelling in nasal passages to relieve stuffiness (e.g., pseudoephedrine, oxymetazoline).

These medications play a key role in managing respiratory conditions, helping people breathe more comfortably and improving their overall quality of life.

6.2. Beta$_2$-Adrenergic Agonists: Breathing Easier

Beta$_2$-adrenergic agonists are commonly prescribed to help people with asthma and chronic obstructive pulmonary disease (COPD) breathe more easily. These medications work by relaxing the muscles around the airways, allowing them to open up and making it easier to inhale and exhale.

There are two main types of beta$_2$-adrenergic agonists:

Short-Acting Beta$_2$-Agonists (SABAs)

These are fast-acting medications used to quickly relieve shortness of breath, wheezing, and chest tightness. They are often referred to as rescue inhalers because they provide immediate relief during an asthma attack or flare-up.

Common short-acting beta$_2$-adrenergic agonists include:

- Albuterol (inhaled, systemic)
- Levalbuterol (inhaled)
- Terbutaline (systemic)

Long-Acting Beta$_2$-Agonists (LABAs)

These medications don't provide immediate relief but help prevent symptoms when used regularly. They are usually prescribed along with inhaled corticosteroids to manage chronic asthma and COPD symptoms over time.

Common long-acting beta$_2$-adrenergic agonists include:

- Formoterol (inhaled)
- Salmeterol (inhaled)
- Arformoterol (inhaled)
- Olodaterol (inhaled)
- Albuterol (oral, systemic) (not commonly used)

Combination Medications

Some inhalers combine a beta$_2$-adrenergic agonist with another medication, such as a steroid or an anticholinergic, to provide better long-term control. Examples include:

- Albuterol and ipratropium (inhalation)
- Budesonide and formoterol (inhalation)
- Formoterol and mometasone (inhalation)
- Salmeterol and fluticasone (inhalation)

How These Medications Work

Beta$_2$-adrenergic agonists help open the airways by relaxing the smooth muscles around them. This process, called bronchodilation, increases airflow to the lungs and makes breathing easier.

- Short-acting inhalers work quickly, making them ideal for sudden breathing problems.
- Long-acting inhalers must be used regularly and are not meant for emergency relief.

How They're Used

Short-Acting Beta$_2$-Agonists (SABAs)

- Best for quick relief during an asthma attack or before exercise (for those with exercise-induced asthma).
- Can be used as needed but should not be overused, as frequent use may indicate poor asthma control.

Long-Acting Beta₂-Agonists (LABAs)

- Used on a fixed schedule to help keep symptoms under control.
- Always prescribed with an anti-inflammatory medication like a steroid to manage chronic inflammation in asthma patients.
- Should never be used as a rescue inhaler during an asthma attack.

Possible Drug Interactions

- Beta-blockers (used for heart conditions) can reduce the effectiveness of beta₂-agonists.
- Certain antidepressants and decongestants may increase the risk of side effects like increased heart rate or tremors.

Side Effects and Precautions

Short-Acting Beta₂-Agonists (SABAs)

- Tremors (shaky hands)
- Fast heartbeat (tachycardia)
- Palpitations (feeling of heart pounding)
- Dry mouth
- Paradoxical bronchospasm (rare, but serious tightening of airways after inhalation)

Long-Acting Beta₂-Agonists (LABAs)

- Increased risk of severe asthma symptoms if used alone without a corticosteroid
- Bronchospasm
- High blood pressure
- Headaches and dizziness

Nursing Considerations and Patient Care

Assessment

- Check respiratory status before and after treatment.
- Monitor peak flow readings to assess lung function.

- Watch for signs of overuse, as excessive use can indicate worsening asthma.

Implementation & Patient Education

- Short-acting inhalers should be used only as needed—overuse can lead to decreased effectiveness over time.
- Long-acting inhalers must be taken daily, even if symptoms are not present.
- Instruct patients to hold their breath for a few seconds after inhalation to allow the medication to work effectively.
- Teach patients to wait at least 2 minutes between inhalations if taking multiple puffs.
- Report worsening symptoms or lack of relief after using a rescue inhaler.

6.3. Anticholinergics: Helping You Breathe Easier

Anticholinergic medications help open the airways by blocking the effects of acetylcholine, a neurotransmitter that causes airway constriction and mucus production. While most oral anticholinergics aren't commonly used for asthma or chronic obstructive pulmonary disease (COPD) due to their tendency to thicken mucus, one inhaled anticholinergic—ipratropium—is frequently used to help manage COPD symptoms.

How Ipratropium Works

Ipratropium relaxes airway muscles by blocking muscarinic receptors in the lungs, allowing air to flow more freely. Unlike $beta_2$-adrenergic agonists (which activate the sympathetic nervous system to open airways), ipratropium prevents airway constriction by inhibiting the parasympathetic nervous system.

Ipratropium can be used alone or in combination with other bronchodilators for better symptom control.

When Is It Used?

Ipratropium is primarily prescribed for:

- COPD patients to prevent wheezing, breathlessness, chest tightness, and coughing.
- Asthma patients as an adjunct therapy (in combination with short-acting beta$_2$-agonists).
- Rhinorrhea (runny nose)—available as a nasal spray for allergy-related nasal congestion.

Important Note: Ipratropium isn't effective for quick relief during an asthma attack. It should not be used as a rescue inhaler for acute bronchospasms.

How the Body Processes It

- Minimal absorption in the bloodstream—mostly works locally in the lungs.
- Metabolized slowly and excreted primarily through urine.
- Does not cross the blood-brain barrier, reducing central nervous system (CNS) side effects.

Possible Drug Interactions

- Generally safe with few interactions, but caution is advised when used with other anticholinergic or antimuscarinic medications as they may increase side effects.

Common Side Effects

Like most medications, ipratropium has some potential side effects, but most are mild.

- Nervousness or dizziness
- Increased heart rate (tachycardia) or palpitations
- Dry mouth (a very common side effect)
- Headache
- Nausea and vomiting

- Constipation or difficulty urinating
- Paradoxical bronchospasm (if overused, can cause airways to tighten instead of opening)

Precaution: If ipratropium accidentally gets into the eyes, it can trigger acute narrow-angle glaucoma, causing blurred vision, eye pain, and increased eye pressure. Patients should close their eyes while using the inhaler to avoid this risk.

Nursing Considerations & Patient Education

Assessment & Monitoring

- Check the patient's breathing pattern before and after starting the medication.
- Monitor peak flow readings to evaluate lung function.
- Watch for signs of worsening symptoms or paradoxical bronchospasm (airway constriction instead of relaxation).

Patient Education

- Don't exceed the recommended doses:
  Inhalation: No more than 12 inhalations per day.
  Nasal spray: No more than 8 sprays per nostril per day.
- If using multiple inhalers, always use the bronchodilator first, wait 5 minutes, then use other inhalers (like steroids).
- Wait 2 minutes between inhalations if taking multiple doses.
- Take on time to maintain effectiveness—don't wait for symptoms to worsen.
- Report worsening symptoms or lack of relief to the healthcare provider.
- Close eyes when inhaling to prevent eye exposure.
- For dry mouth, patients can chew gum, suck on ice chips, or stay hydrated.

6.4. Corticosteroids & Leukotriene Modifiers: Managing Inflammation & Asthma

Corticosteroids and leukotriene modifiers play a crucial role in controlling asthma and other inflammatory conditions. They help prevent exacerbations, reduce airway inflammation, and improve long-term respiratory health.

Corticosteroids: The Powerhouses of Anti-Inflammation

Corticosteroids are some of the most effective anti-inflammatory drugs for asthma management. They come in three forms, depending on how they're administered:

1. Inhaled Corticosteroids (ICS) – Daily Prevention

Used long-term to reduce airway inflammation, helping prevent asthma symptoms. Common ICS include:

- Beclomethasone
- Budesonide
- Fluticasone
- Mometasone

2. Oral Corticosteroids – Short-Term Control

These are stronger and used for asthma flare-ups or severe inflammation:

- Prednisone
- Prednisolone

3. IV Corticosteroids – Emergency Treatment

Given in the hospital during severe asthma attacks:

- Dexamethasone

- Methylprednisolone

How Corticosteroids Work

- Block inflammatory mediators like cytokines & prostaglandins.
- Prevent immune cells (like eosinophils) from causing airway inflammation.
- Reduce mucus production and swelling in the lungs.
- Enhance the effects of bronchodilators, making breathing easier.

Not for quick relief! Corticosteroids don't work immediately—they're preventative, not rescue medications.

Possible Side Effects

Inhaled Corticosteroids

- Mild – Hoarseness, cough, throat irritation.
- Common – Oral thrush (candida infection in the mouth).

Prevention Tip: Rinse your mouth after using an inhaled steroid!

Oral & IV Corticosteroids (Short-Term)

- Increased blood sugar – Caution in diabetics.
- Insomnia, mood swings, headaches – Can be bothersome.
- Nausea, upset stomach – Take with food to minimize discomfort.

Oral & IV Corticosteroids (Long-Term)

Serious risks if used for months/years:

- Osteoporosis & bone fractures.
- Growth suppression in children.
- Weight gain & fluid retention.
- Weakened immune system – Higher infection risk.

Never stop corticosteroids suddenly! Tapering is necessary to avoid withdrawal symptoms & adrenal insufficiency.

Best Practices for Taking Corticosteroids

- Inhaled steroids – Use a spacer to prevent oral thrush.
- Oral steroids – Take with food to prevent stomach issues.
- Long-term use? Monitor bone density, blood sugar, & weight.
- Wash hands & avoid sick people – Your immune system might be weaker.

Leukotriene Modifiers: An Alternative for Asthma Prevention

What Are They?

Leukotriene modifiers are not steroids—they work by blocking leukotrienes, inflammatory chemicals that cause swelling, mucus, and bronchoconstriction in asthma.

They are used daily for asthma prevention, not for immediate relief.

Types of Leukotriene Modifiers

Leukotriene Receptor Blockers – Stop leukotrienes from binding to receptors:

- Montelukast (Singulair)
- Zafirlukast (Accolate)

Leukotriene Formation Inhibitors – Prevent leukotrienes from forming:

- Zileuton (Zyflo)

How They Work

- Prevent asthma symptoms by blocking airway inflammation.
- Reduce airway swelling & mucus production.
- Improve lung function over time.
- Help patients reduce reliance on steroids.

Not for quick relief! They don't stop an asthma attack—they prevent future flare-ups.

Possible Side Effects

- Mild – Headache, nausea, dizziness.
- Rare but serious – Mood changes, aggression, suicidal thoughts (especially in children).

Monitor mood & behavior, especially in kids!

Best Practices for Taking Leukotriene Modifiers

- Take daily, even if you feel fine – It prevents symptoms, but doesn't work instantly.
- Zafirlukast – Take on an empty stomach (food reduces absorption).
- Montelukast – Can be taken with or without food.
- Monitor liver function if using Zileuton, as it can affect liver enzymes.

6.5. Mast Cell Stabilizers: Preventing Asthma & Allergies Naturally

Mast cell stabilizers help prevent asthma symptoms and control long-term inflammation, especially in children and those with mild asthma. These medications are not for quick relief during an asthma attack but work to reduce airway sensitivity over time.

What Are Mast Cell Stabilizers?

These non-steroidal anti-inflammatory drugs help control asthma and allergic reactions by stopping mast cells (a type of immune cell) from releasing inflammatory chemicals.

Common Mast Cell Stabilizer:

- Cromolyn sodium – Available as inhalers, nasal sprays, and eye drops.

How They Work

- Stabilize mast cells – Prevent the release of histamines & inflammatory mediators.

- Reduce airway inflammation – Makes the lungs less sensitive to triggers.
- Control allergic reactions – Helpful for asthma caused by allergens.
- Great for exercise-induced asthma – Can be taken before exercise to prevent symptoms.

Mast cell stabilizers are preventatives! They must be used regularly to be effective—not for quick relief during an asthma attack.

Best Uses for Mast Cell Stabilizers

- Mild persistent asthma – Reduces inflammation over time.
- Exercise-induced asthma – Take before physical activity to prevent symptoms.
- Seasonal allergies (hay fever) – Available as nasal sprays & eye drops to reduce allergy symptoms.

Not effective for emergency asthma attacks! Use a rescue inhaler (albuterol) for immediate relief.

Possible Side Effects

Mast cell stabilizers are generally well tolerated, but some people may experience:

- Mild effects – Cough, throat irritation, headache.
- Rare effects – Wheezing, bronchospasm (tightening of airways).

Tip: If symptoms worsen after inhaling, use a bronchodilator first to open airways before taking the mast cell stabilizer.

Best Practices for Taking Mast Cell Stabilizers

- Take regularly – Effects build over 1-2 weeks (not instant).
- For exercise-induced asthma – Use 15-30 minutes before exercise.
- For allergies – Use nasal spray or eye drops as directed.
- Use a spacer with inhalers to reduce throat irritation.

6.6. Methylxanthines: Breathing Easier with Theophylline & Aminophylline

Methylxanthines, also known as xanthines, are used to treat asthma, chronic bronchitis, and emphysema. While they aren't the first choice for managing breathing problems, they can be helpful when other medications don't work.

What Are Methylxanthines?

These drugs relax airway muscles and improve breathing by reducing airway inflammation and increasing respiratory drive.

Common Methylxanthines:

- Aminophylline – Used IV for severe cases.
- Theophylline – Most commonly used oral form.

Methylxanthines aren't quick-relief drugs! They work best for long-term control and are not meant to replace a rescue inhaler (albuterol).

How Do They Work?

- Relax airway muscles – Makes breathing easier.
- Reduce inflammation – Less mucus & airway swelling.
- Stimulate respiratory drive – Helps the brain breathe more efficiently in conditions like COPD.
- Improve diaphragm function – Reduces fatigue in chronic lung diseases.

Toxicity risk is a concern! The therapeutic range for theophylline is 10-20 mcg/mL, and levels must be monitored to avoid side effects.

When Are They Used?

- Asthma – For long-term symptom control.
- Chronic bronchitis & emphysema – Helps keep airways open.
- Neonatal apnea – Used in premature babies with breathing problems.

These drugs are usually considered "second-line" treatments—they're used when inhalers and other medications don't fully control symptoms.

Drug Interactions

Methylxanthines interact with many medications, so they must be carefully monitored:

Drugs that increase theophylline levels (higher toxicity risk):

- Antibiotics: Erythromycin, clarithromycin, ciprofloxacin
- Heart medications: Verapamil, diltiazem
- Hormonal contraceptives
- Antifungals: Ketoconazole, fluconazole

Drugs that lower theophylline levels (less effective medication):

- Seizure meds: Phenytoin, carbamazepine, phenobarbital
- Smoking (cigarettes or marijuana) – Increases drug breakdown

Caffeine (coffee, tea, sodas) can worsen side effects! Avoid drinking large amounts while on this medication.

Side Effects to Watch For

Methylxanthines can cause temporary side effects or toxicity if blood levels get too high.

Mild Side Effects

- Nausea, vomiting, diarrhea
- Headache, dizziness
- Restlessness, trouble sleeping

Signs of Toxicity (Too Much Drug in the Blood)

- Severe nausea & vomiting
- Fast or irregular heartbeat
- Seizures
- Confusion or shakiness

If toxicity occurs, the drug should be stopped immediately, and medical attention is needed!

Best Practices for Taking Methylxanthines

- Take at the same time each day for steady blood levels.
- Avoid caffeine to prevent overstimulation.
- Smokers may need higher doses – Smoking speeds up drug breakdown.
- Elderly & liver patients need lower doses – Their bodies process the drug more slowly.
- Regular blood tests are needed to prevent toxicity!
- Never crush or chew extended-release tablets!

6.7. Expectorants: Helping You Breathe Easier

When you're dealing with chest congestion and a stubborn cough, expectorants like guaifenesin can help loosen up mucus, making it easier to clear your airways. They don't stop a cough—they make it more productive, so you can get rid of excess mucus more efficiently.

What Are Expectorants?

Expectorants increase bronchial secretions, thin mucus, and help clear airways. The most commonly used expectorant is guaifenesin, which is found in many over-the-counter (OTC) cold and flu medications.

How Does Guaifenesin Work?

- Increases fluid in the respiratory tract – Thins out thick, sticky mucus.
- Soothes the airway lining – Helps reduce irritation.
- Makes coughing more effective – Instead of a dry, hacking cough, mucus is cleared out more easily.

Expectorants work best when taken with plenty of water! 💧 Staying hydrated helps thin the mucus even more, making it easier to expel.

When Is It Used?

Guaifenesin is used to relieve congestion and help clear mucus in conditions like:

- Colds & flu
- Bronchitis
- Sinus infections
- Asthma-related mucus buildup
- Emphysema & minor bronchial irritation

Expectorants are NOT cough suppressants! If your goal is to stop coughing, you may need a cough suppressant like dextromethorphan instead.

Are There Any Drug Interactions?

There are no major drug interactions with guaifenesin. However, it's often combined with other medications (like decongestants or cough suppressants), so always check the label before taking multiple cold and flu medications.

Possible Side Effects

Most people tolerate guaifenesin well, but some may experience mild side effects, especially with high doses:

Common Side Effects:

- Nausea, vomiting (if taken in large amounts)
- Diarrhea
- Drowsiness
- Abdominal pain
- Headache
- Skin rash or hives (rare)

If a rash or allergic reaction occurs, stop taking the medication and seek medical attention!

Best Practices for Taking Expectorants

- Drink plenty of water to help loosen mucus.
- Take as directed, with a full glass of water.
- Use a humidifier to keep airways moist.
- Avoid unnecessary medications – Don't mix with other OTC drugs unless approved by a doctor or pharmacist.
- Report a lingering cough – If symptoms last longer than 7 days or get worse, consult a healthcare provider.

6.8. Understanding Antitussives: When and How to Use Them for Cough Relief

When a persistent, dry cough keeps you up at night or interferes with your daily activities, antitussives (cough suppressants) can help. Unlike expectorants, which help clear mucus, antitussives work by reducing the urge to cough, making them ideal for nonproductive coughs that are irritating and exhausting.

What Are Antitussives?

Antitussives work by suppressing the cough reflex, helping you rest and recover. Common antitussive medications include:

- Benzonatate – Numbs the cough reflex in the airways.
- Dextromethorphan (DM) – The most widely used OTC cough suppressant.
- Codeine – A mild opioid, often prescribed for severe, persistent coughs.
- Hydrocodone – A stronger opioid for intractable coughs that don't respond to other treatments.

Antitussives are best used for dry, hacking coughs that aren't bringing up mucus. If you have a productive cough, an expectorant like guaifenesin may be a better choice!

How Do Antitussives Work?

Different types of antitussives work in different ways:

- Benzonatate: Numbs the throat and lungs, reducing the urge to cough.
- Dextromethorphan, Codeine, and Hydrocodone: Suppress the cough reflex by acting directly on the brain's cough center.

Opioid antitussives (like codeine & hydrocodone) should only be used for severe coughs and under medical supervision due to the risk of dependence.

When Are They Used?

Antitussives help relieve persistent, dry coughs caused by:

- Colds & flu
- Bronchitis
- Pneumonia (only for dry cough)
- Chronic lung conditions like COPD or emphysema
- Postnasal drip
- Allergies

They should NOT be used for coughs that bring up mucus, as this can trap phlegm in the lungs and lead to infections.

Possible Drug Interactions

Some medications don't mix well with antitussives. Be cautious when combining:

Opioid antitussives (Codeine, Hydrocodone):

- Avoid combining with alcohol, sedatives, or sleeping aids – This can increase drowsiness and slow breathing.
- Don't use with monoamine oxidase inhibitors (MAOIs) – May cause dangerously high blood pressure or coma.

Dextromethorphan:

- Shouldn't be taken with SSRIs (like fluoxetine or sertraline) – May lead to a rare but serious reaction called serotonin syndrome.

Always check with a doctor or pharmacist before taking antitussives with other medications!

Possible Side Effects

Benzonatate Side Effects:

- Dizziness, drowsiness
- Mouth & throat numbness (if chewed)
- Nasal congestion
- GI discomfort (nausea, constipation)

Benzonatate capsules should NEVER be chewed or crushed! This can numb the throat, leading to choking or difficulty swallowing.

Opioid Antitussive Side Effects (Codeine, Hydrocodone):

- Drowsiness, dizziness
- Nausea & vomiting
- Constipation
- Slowed breathing (in high doses)
- Potential for dependence or addiction

Use opioid-based cough suppressants only as prescribed, and never in children under 18 without a doctor's approval.

Best Practices for Taking Antitussives

- Take as directed – Stick to the correct dose and timing.
- Drink plenty of fluids – Keeps the throat moist and helps relieve irritation.
- Avoid alcohol & sedatives – Especially with opioid-based medications.
- Use only when needed – Don't suppress a productive cough unless necessary.
- Watch for worsening symptoms – If your cough lasts more than 7 days, or if you have fever, chest pain, or trouble breathing, seek medical advice.

6.9.   Decongestants: How They Work and When to Use Them

If you're dealing with nasal congestion from a cold, allergies, or sinus infection, decongestants can help shrink swollen nasal passages, making it easier to breathe. These medications relieve stuffy noses by reducing swelling and increasing airflow in the nasal passages.

What Are Decongestants?

Decongestants come in two forms:

- Systemic Decongestants (Oral) – Work throughout the body to shrink swollen blood vessels in the nose.
- Topical Decongestants (Nasal Sprays or Drops) – Act directly in the nose to provide fast relief.

Common Decongestants

Systemic (Oral) Decongestants:

- Pseudoephedrine (Sudafed) – Most effective oral decongestant
- Phenylephrine – Found in many OTC cold medicines
- Ephedrine – Used in some prescription medications

Topical (Nasal Spray or Drops) Decongestants:

- Oxymetazoline (Afrin, Dristan) – Works fast, but shouldn't be used more than 3 days
- Phenylephrine – Also available as a nasal spray
- Naphazoline, Tetrahydrozoline – Less commonly used

Which is better? Nasal sprays provide quicker relief but can cause rebound congestion if used for too long. Oral decongestants last longer but may have more side effects.

How Do Decongestants Work?

- Shrink swollen blood vessels in the nose, reducing congestion
- Improve sinus drainage and relieve pressure

- Open blocked eustachian tubes (which can help relieve ear pressure)

Important: Decongestants don't cure colds or allergies—they only relieve symptoms!

When to Use Decongestants

Decongestants help clear up nasal congestion caused by:

- Colds & Flu
- Allergies (Hay Fever)
- Sinus Infections
- Vasomotor Rhinitis (non-allergic nasal inflammation)

If your congestion is due to allergies, an antihistamine may work better—or you may need to combine both.

Potential Drug Interactions & Warnings

Avoid Decongestants If You Have:

- High Blood Pressure – Can raise blood pressure even more
- Glaucoma – Can increase eye pressure
- Heart Disease – Can put extra strain on the heart
- Diabetes – May affect blood sugar levels
- Hyperthyroidism – Can worsen symptoms
- Enlarged Prostate (BPH) – Can make urination more difficult

Drug Interactions:

- Avoid using decongestants with MAO inhibitors (like phenelzine or selegiline) – Can cause dangerous blood pressure spikes.
- Be cautious if taking stimulant medications (ADHD meds, caffeine, etc.) – Can increase heart rate.
- Don't mix with other cold medications without checking labels – Many OTC products contain hidden decongestants!

Side Effects of Decongestants

Systemic (Oral) Decongestants:

Can cause:

- Increased heart rate (palpitations, tachycardia)
- Nervousness or anxiety
- Insomnia
- Dizziness
- Increased blood pressure

Topical (Nasal) Decongestants:

Can cause:

- Rebound congestion if used for more than 3 days
- Burning or stinging sensation in the nose
- Dry nasal passages

To avoid rebound congestion, use nasal sprays for no more than 3 consecutive days!

Best Practices for Using Decongestants

- Oral decongestants: Take with a full glass of water, avoid before bedtime to prevent insomnia.
- Nasal sprays: Use for 3 days MAX to avoid rebound congestion.
- Monitor blood pressure: If you have hypertension, talk to your doctor before using decongestants.
- Stay hydrated: Decongestants can dry out nasal passages—drink extra fluids.

If your congestion lasts more than 10 days, or if you have fever, facial pain, or swelling, seek medical attention—it may be a sinus infection.

Chapter 7: Gastrointestinal Medicines

7.1. Understanding GI Medications

The gastrointestinal (GI) system is like a complex processing plant—it digests food, absorbs nutrients, and gets rid of waste. When something goes wrong, it can cause pain, bloating, acid reflux, diarrhea, constipation, or nausea. Thankfully, there are many medications that help regulate digestion and relieve discomfort.

What Are GI Medications?

Different classes of GI medications target specific digestive issues:

- Antiulcer Drugs – Help heal and prevent stomach ulcers, acid reflux, and heartburn.
- Adsorbents & Antiflatulents – Reduce gas and bloating.
- Digestive Enzymes – Help break down food for better absorption.
- Antidiarrheal Medications – Slow down frequent or loose stools.
- Laxatives – Relieve constipation by promoting bowel movements.
- Obesity Medications – Assist with weight loss and appetite control.
- Antiemetic Drugs – Help prevent or stop nausea and vomiting.

Each of these drug types plays a unique role in keeping your digestive system balanced and functioning properly.

Things to Consider When Using GI Medications

- Read the labels – Some GI medications can interact with other drugs.

- Monitor side effects – Many over-the-counter (OTC) and prescription GI drugs can cause mild side effects like dizziness, bloating, or dry mouth.
- Short-term vs. Long-term use – Some medications (like laxatives and acid reducers) shouldn't be overused to avoid dependency or worsening symptoms.

When to See a Doctor:

- Severe or persistent symptoms that don't improve after taking GI medications
- Blood in your stool or vomit
- Unexplained weight loss or difficulty swallowing

Your digestive health is key to your overall well-being! Understanding these medications can help you take control of your gut health.

7.2. Antiulcer Drugs – Healing the Gut, One Dose at a Time

Peptic ulcers are painful sores that develop in the lining of the stomach, lower esophagus, or small intestine (usually the duodenum). They occur when acid and digestive enzymes break down the protective lining of your digestive tract faster than it can repair itself.

What Causes Ulcers?

Several things can tip the balance in your gut and lead to ulcer formation:

- H. pylori infection – A common bacteria that disrupts the stomach's defense barrier.
- NSAIDs – Regular use of medications like ibuprofen or aspirin.
- Zollinger-Ellison syndrome – A rare condition that causes excessive acid production.
- Smoking – Increases acid secretion and slows healing.
- Genetics – Ulcers can run in families.

How Antiulcer Medications Work

Antiulcer drugs either kill the bacteria, neutralize or reduce stomach acid, or protect the lining of your stomach and intestines. Common categories include:

1. Systemic Antibiotics

If H. pylori is the cause, antibiotics are essential to wipe out the infection. Doctors usually prescribe a combination of two antibiotics, often alongside a proton pump inhibitor (PPI) or H2 blocker, to fully heal the ulcer and prevent it from returning.

Common antibiotics used:

- Amoxicillin
- Clarithromycin
- Metronidazole
- Tetracycline

Things to know:

- Food affects absorption, especially dairy with tetracycline.
- Adverse effects may include GI upset, metallic taste (with metronidazole), or diarrhea.
- Don't mix alcohol with metronidazole—it can cause a nasty reaction.

2. Antacids

These are your fast-acting, over-the-counter relief heroes. Antacids neutralize stomach acid and soothe that burning pain of heartburn or indigestion. They don't treat the cause of ulcers, but they do bring temporary comfort.

Types include:

- Calcium carbonate
- Magnesium hydroxide
- Aluminum hydroxide

- Magaldrate
- Simethicone

Watch out for:

- Constipation (with aluminum/calcium-based antacids)
- Diarrhea (with magnesium-based ones)
- Electrolyte imbalances with long-term use
- Interference with other medications—separate by at least 2 hours.

3. H2-Receptor Antagonists

Often referred to as "H2 blockers," these drugs reduce acid production by blocking histamine at specific stomach receptors.

Common examples:

- Cimetidine
- Ranitidine (note: many brands withdrawn from market)
- Famotidine
- Nizatidine

Why use them? They're great for treating:

- Active ulcers
- GERD
- Reflux esophagitis
- Preventing ulcers in critically ill patients

Side effects to watch for:

- Headaches, dizziness, fatigue
- Cimetidine may cause gynecomastia (breast enlargement in men), libido loss, and drug interactions
- Elderly patients or those with kidney/liver issues may be more sensitive

Timing tip: Give H2 blockers at bedtime for once-a-day dosing. If prescribed twice daily, give one dose in the morning and one in the evening.

Putting It All Together

Peptic ulcer treatment usually involves a combination of medications tailored to your cause—especially if H. pylori is involved. Treatment often includes:

- Two antibiotics
- A PPI or H2 blocker
- Possibly an antacid for symptom relief

Treatment usually lasts 2 weeks, with acid-suppressing therapy continuing for another 4 to 6 weeks to ensure complete healing.

Nursing Care and Patient Guidance

Assessment

- Monitor ulcer symptoms and signs of H. pylori infection.
- Watch for adverse reactions—especially GI distress, allergic reactions, or fluid imbalances.
- Identify risk factors like smoking, NSAID use, or stress.

Nursing Diagnoses

- Risk for fluid imbalance due to GI symptoms
- Ineffective health maintenance
- Knowledge deficit about medication use

Goals

- Reduced or eliminated ulcer symptoms
- Stable vital signs and improved hydration
- Understanding of the treatment plan and proper medication use

Implementation Tips

- Always take the full course of antibiotics, even if you feel better early.
- Separate antacids from other drugs by 1-2 hours.
- Monitor for signs of electrolyte imbalance or drug interactions.
- Encourage patients to avoid smoking, limit alcohol, and manage stress.

Evaluation

- Patient reports reduced pain or burning.
- Normal lab results (electrolytes, kidney function, CBC).
- Patient can explain why and how to take their medications.

Proton Pump Inhibitors (PPIs): Turning Down the Acid

When your stomach's acid production gets out of hand, proton pump inhibitors (PPIs) step in to calm things down. They block the final step of acid secretion in the stomach, helping ulcers heal and easing irritation.

Common PPIs include:

- Dexlansoprazole
- Esomeprazole
- Lansoprazole
- Omeprazole
- Pantoprazole
- Rabeprazole

How They Work in Your Body

- Given by mouth, usually as enteric-coated tablets or capsules (so the stomach acid doesn't break them down too soon).
- Absorbed in the small intestine and processed by the liver before being flushed out in the urine.

- Some (like esomeprazole and pantoprazole) can also be given by IV in hospital settings.

PPIs stop acid production by targeting the hydrogen-potassium ATPase enzyme (aka the "proton pump") in the stomach lining's parietal cells—the source of that excess acid.

Why They're Prescribed

- Healing gastric or duodenal ulcers
- Treating GERD and erosive esophagitis
- Reducing acid in Zollinger-Ellison syndrome (a rare condition with overactive acid production)
- Fighting H. pylori infections (alongside antibiotics)
- Managing chronic hyperacidic conditions

Drug Interactions to Watch

- PPIs can slow down the breakdown of drugs like warfarin, diazepam, and phenytoin—increasing their effects.
- They may also reduce absorption of certain nutrients or medications that need stomach acid to work properly (e.g., calcium, iron, magnesium, vitamin B12, ketoconazole).

Potential Side Effects

- Nausea, vomiting, abdominal pain, and gas

Long-term use may lead to:

- Osteoporosis-related fractures
- Clostridium difficile infections
- Low magnesium levels
- Increased pneumonia risk

Nursing Tips for PPIs

Assessment:

- Monitor for side effects and potential drug interactions.

- Keep an eye on fluid balance, especially if GI symptoms occur.

Key Diagnoses:

- Impaired tissue integrity (due to ulcers)
- Risk for fluid volume deficit (from GI effects)
- Knowledge deficit (about meds and side effects)

Goals:

- Reduced ulcer pain and acid symptoms
- Maintained hydration and stable vitals
- Understanding and adherence to drug plan

Implementation:

- Give PPIs 30 minutes before meals.
- Do not crush or chew capsules—swallow whole.
- If given IV, check hospital policy for correct reconstitution and infusion instructions.

Evaluation:

- Patient experiences relief from symptoms.
- Patient maintains good hydration.
- Patient and family understand how to take the medication safely.

Other Antiulcer Drugs: Misoprostol & Sucralfate

Sometimes, patients need more targeted help, especially if NSAIDs or stress are contributing to ulcers. Two other medications that provide protection are:

Misoprostol (Cytotec)

A synthetic prostaglandin E1, misoprostol reduces acid and increases protective mucus in the stomach.

- Given orally, metabolized quickly, and eliminated in urine.
- Used to prevent NSAID-related ulcers.

- Not safe in pregnancy—can cause miscarriage.

Common side effects: Diarrhea, gas, nausea, abdominal pain

Sucralfate (Carafate)

Think of sucralfate as a protective bandage for your stomach. It forms a sticky paste that clings to ulcers, shielding them from acid while they heal.

- Works only in the stomach (not absorbed into the bloodstream).
- Often used for short-term ulcer treatment or ulcer prevention.

Common side effects: Constipation, nausea, a metallic taste

How to Use Them

Misoprostol:

- Take with meals.
- Women of childbearing age should use reliable contraception and start the drug after the second or third day of menstruation to avoid unintended pregnancy.

Sucralfate:

- Take it 1 hour before meals and at bedtime.
- Avoid taking antacids within 30 minutes, as they reduce its effectiveness.

Nursing Process for Misoprostol & Sucralfate

Assessment:

- Monitor for GI symptoms and adverse effects.
- In women: verify non-pregnancy status and discuss contraception.

Key Diagnoses:

- Impaired tissue integrity
- Fluid volume deficit (from GI symptoms)

- Knowledge deficit

Goals:

- Symptom relief and ulcer healing
- No dehydration or GI complications
- Understanding safe use of therapy

Implementation:

- Stress importance of continuing therapy at home, even if symptoms improve early.
- Recommend avoiding triggers like smoking, alcohol, spicy foods, and large meals before bedtime.
- Elevate the head of the bed for comfort.

Evaluation:

- Symptoms are under control
- Adequate fluid intake
- Patient and family can explain the purpose and use of the meds

7.3. Helping the Gut: Adsorbents, Antiflatulents, and Digestive Drugs

These medications support a healthier gastrointestinal (GI) system by addressing toxins, gas buildup, and digestion issues. Let's break down what they do and when they're used.

Adsorbent Drugs: Blocking the Bad Stuff

What they're for:

Adsorbents are often used in emergency situations when someone swallows something toxic. They trap harmful substances in the gut before they can be absorbed into the bloodstream.

Main player:

Activated charcoal – a black powder made from organic materials. It's the go-to antidote for many types of poisoning.

How it works:

It binds to toxins still in the stomach or intestines and carries them out through the stool. It doesn't work if the substance has already been absorbed, and it's not effective against things like alcohol, acids, or metals.

Special tip: Sometimes, toxins get reabsorbed through the intestines after being processed by the liver. Giving repeated doses of activated charcoal helps break this cycle.

Side effects:

- Black stools (totally normal)
- Constipation (a laxative is often given with it)

Nursing Notes for Adsorbents

Assessment:

- Find out what substance was ingested and when.
- Watch for constipation or vomiting.
- Check if the patient (especially children or post-surgery) is at risk for GI obstruction or complications.

Implementation:

- Mix charcoal with water until syrupy. Flavoring helps with taste, but no milk or ice cream!
- Only give to conscious patients or through an NG tube.
- Keep emergency equipment nearby—just in case.

Evaluation:

- Patient avoids harm from the toxin.
- Fluid levels stay stable.
- Patient and caregivers understand what the drug does.

Antiflatulent Drugs: Fighting the Bloat

What they're for:

Antiflatulents help relieve the discomfort of gas by breaking it up so it can pass more easily.

Star of the show:

Simethicone – found in many OTC gas relief meds.

How it works:

Simethicone reduces surface tension, popping gas bubbles in the intestines and helping the body get rid of them more comfortably.

Used for:

- Bloating
- Post-surgery gas
- Diverticular disease
- Air swallowing (yes, that's a thing)

Side effects:

- None known—maybe just some extra belching or flatus (but that's kind of the goal!).

Nursing Notes for Antiflatulents

Assessment:

- Ask about gas pain, bloating, or discomfort.
- Check for any other digestive issues.

Implementation:

- Make sure chewables are actually chewed.
- Shake liquid suspensions before giving.
- Encourage movement—walking helps release gas.

- Less bloating and gas.
- Patient understands how and when to use the medication.

Digestive Drugs: Helping the Body Break It Down

What they're for:

These drugs help people who can't properly digest food due to missing enzymes or bile acids.

Examples:

- Dehydrocholic acid – boosts bile production
- Pancreatic enzymes (like pancrelipase) – replace digestive enzymes for fats, carbs, and proteins

Who needs them?

- People with chronic pancreatitis, cystic fibrosis, pancreatic cancer, or those who've had certain stomach surgeries
- Also used to treat steatorrhea (fatty stools)

How they work:

They mimic the natural digestive substances the body usually makes and act locally in the intestines (they're not absorbed into the bloodstream).

Side effects:

- Abdominal cramps
- Diarrhea or nausea
- If bile ducts are blocked, bile acid drugs may cause colic

Nursing Notes for Digestive Drugs

Assessment:

- Watch for changes in digestion, weight, or bowel habits.

- Monitor how well the patient tolerates fats and proteins in their diet.
- Check for knowledge gaps in drug use or nutrition.

Implementation:

- Give enzymes before or with meals.
- For kids, you can mix powdered forms with applesauce.
- Don't crush enteric-coated capsules—open and sprinkle if needed, but always follow with a drink.
- Offer support with food preferences and dietary restrictions. Bring in a dietitian if needed.

Evaluation:

- Normal digestion of fats, carbs, and proteins
- Good compliance with meds and diet
- Patient and family understand the purpose and use of the drugs

7.4. Balancing Bowel Function: Antidiarrheals & Laxatives

Digestive health is all about balance—and when the large intestine gets out of rhythm, we see two extremes: diarrhea and constipation. Fortunately, there are medications that can help restore normal bowel patterns and comfort.

Let's take a look at the different types of medications used to manage these symptoms.

Antidiarrheals: Slowing Things Down

These drugs help control loose, frequent bowel movements. Some work systemically (throughout the body), while others act directly in the gut.

Opioid-Related Antidiarrheals

Common examples:

- Diphenoxylate with atropine
- Loperamide (Imodium)

How they work:

These medications slow down the movement of the intestines (peristalsis), giving the body more time to absorb fluids and firm up the stool.

How they move through the body:

- Diphenoxylate is well absorbed, while loperamide isn't absorbed much at all.
- Both are broken down in the liver and mostly leave the body in stool.

What they treat:

- Sudden (acute) or ongoing (chronic) diarrhea that's not caused by infection.

Possible side effects:

- **Nausea, vomiting, abdominal cramps**
- Drowsiness or fatigue
- Rare but serious: slowed breathing, fast heart rate, or even bowel obstruction (paralytic ileus)

Nursing Tips:

- Always assess hydration, bowel patterns, and possible infection before giving.
- Encourage fluids!
- Watch for side effects like drowsiness or dehydration.
- Teach patients to follow exact dosing and not to double up if a dose is missed.

Kaolin & Pectin: The Gentle Soothers

These over-the-counter remedies work right in the gut to absorb toxins and calm irritation. Think of them as a "sponge" for your digestive tract.

How they work:

- Kaolin binds to bacteria and toxins.
- Pectin lowers gut pH and soothes inflammation.

Used for:

- Mild to moderate diarrhea or to temporarily calm chronic symptoms.

Watch out for:

- Constipation, especially in older or weakened patients.
- Reduced absorption of other medications (don't take them together!).

Laxatives: Getting Things Moving

When constipation strikes, these medications help the body eliminate stool. There are several types, depending on how they work.

Hyperosmolar Laxatives

These draw water into the intestines to soften stool and trigger movement.

Common types:

- Glycerin (suppository or enema)
- Lactulose
- PEG (polyethylene glycol) – gentle and commonly used for bowel prep
- Saline compounds – like magnesium citrate or sodium phosphate

What they treat:

- Constipation (regular or severe)
- Bowel retraining
- High ammonia levels in liver disease (lactulose)

Possible side effects:

- Cramping, gas, diarrhea
- Dehydration or electrolyte imbalances (especially with saline types)
- Rare: heart rhythm issues or blood pressure drops (in vulnerable patients)

Nursing Process Across These Drugs

Assessment

- Get a baseline on bowel habits, hydration, and symptoms.
- Track intake/output and stool patterns.
- Look for signs of dehydration or electrolyte imbalance.

Implementation

- Follow timing instructions—some drugs need to be taken before meals or bedtime.
- Don't crush coated tablets.
- Ensure easy bathroom access.
- Encourage fiber, hydration, and movement to prevent future constipation.

Goals & Outcomes

- Patient achieves regular bowel movements.
- Hydration and electrolyte levels stay stable.
- Patient feels less pain and understands how to use their medication properly.

Dietary Fiber & Bulk-Forming Laxatives: Going the Natural Route

The most natural way to prevent or manage constipation? Good old dietary fiber. It's the part of plants that your small intestine can't digest—and that's a good thing.

Mimicking Nature

Bulk-forming laxatives are made to behave like dietary fiber. These include:

- Methylcellulose
- Polycarbophil
- Psyllium hydrophilic mucilloid

How They Work

These agents aren't absorbed into the bloodstream. Instead, your gut bacteria help break them down into compounds that draw water into the intestines. This softens the stool and increases bulk, nudging your gut to get moving again.

Why They're Used

Bulk-forming laxatives can:

- Treat basic constipation, especially due to low fiber or fluid intake
- Help patients who shouldn't strain (like after a heart attack or aneurysm)
- Manage symptoms of IBS or diverticulosis

Important Drug Interactions

They can reduce absorption of certain meds like digoxin, warfarin, and aspirin if taken too close together. Leave at least a two-hour gap.

Potential Side Effects

- Gas and bloating

- A sense of fullness
- Intestinal blockage or even fecal impaction (especially if not taken with enough fluids)
- Rarely, esophageal obstruction or diarrhea

Nursing Considerations

- Monitor bowel movements, stool consistency, and GI symptoms.
- Encourage adequate fluid intake and activity.
- Mix powdered forms well with water or soft food—never give dry powder alone.
- Laxative effects typically kick in within 12–24 hours but may take up to 3 days.

Emollient Laxatives (Stool Softeners): Gentle Relief

These are your go-to for patients who should avoid straining. Options include:

- Docusate calcium
- Docusate potassium
- Docusate sodium

How They Work

They help fat and water mix into stool, softening it. They also encourage the intestines to release more water and electrolytes into the stool, making it easier to pass.

Who Needs Them

Great for patients:

- Post-surgery or post-MI
- With anorectal conditions
- With increased ICP or hernias

Caution

Avoid taking them with mineral oil, which can be absorbed into tissues—leading to unwanted complications.

Possible Side Effects

- Bitter taste
- Diarrhea or cramping
- Mild throat irritation

Nursing Considerations

- Shake suspensions well and give with water.
- Make sure the patient has bathroom access.
- Educate patients on lifestyle measures to prevent constipation.

Stimulant Laxatives: Fast-Track Bowel Movements

These include:

- Bisacodyl
- Cascara sagrada
- Castor oil
- Phenolphthalein
- Senna

How They Work

These irritate the intestinal lining or stimulate nerves to trigger strong peristalsis. Castor oil also targets the small intestine directly.

Common Uses

Ideal for:

- Pre-surgical bowel prep
- Pre-colonoscopy or barium studies
- Constipation from inactivity, nerve dysfunction, or opioids

Watch for

- Cramping
- Nausea
- Weakness
- Rectal discomfort
- Discolored urine (with senna or cascara)

Pro Tip

Avoid giving them with other oral meds at the same time—they can interfere with absorption.

Lubricant Laxatives: The Smooth Operator

Mineral oil is the main player here.

How It Works

It coats the stool and intestinal lining, locking in moisture and preventing water reabsorption. This leads to easier passage. When given rectally, it also stretches the rectum, promoting the urge to go.

Who It's For

- Patients recovering from MI, eye surgery, or aneurysm repair
- Those with fecal impaction

Be Careful With

- Interference with nutrient and medication absorption, especially vitamins A, D, E, K, oral contraceptives, and anticoagulants

Side Effects

- Nausea and vomiting
- Diarrhea or cramping

Nursing Considerations

- Give oral doses on an empty stomach.
- Administer enemas according to protocol.

- Time doses to avoid disrupting sleep or daily routine.

General Laxative Nursing Considerations

Assessment:

- Get a good GI history and baseline bowel habits
- Monitor bowel movements, stool appearance, and patient comfort
- Check for hydration and electrolyte balance

Planning Goals:

- Regular, easy bowel movements
- Minimal pain or cramping
- Clear understanding of how and when to use medications

Implementation:

- Make sure patients are well hydrated
- Encourage movement and fiber intake
- Don't crush enteric-coated pills
- Time meds to avoid interfering with sleep or daily life
- Provide bathroom access

Evaluation:

- Is the patient having regular bowel movements?
- Is pain gone?
- Does the patient (and caregiver) understand how to manage constipation safely?

Medications for Chronic Constipation and IBS

Chronic constipation isn't just the occasional sluggish bowel—it's defined as constipation that sticks around for six months or more. It's especially common in people with irritable bowel syndrome with constipation (IBS-C).

Chloride Channel Activator

Lubiprostone (Amitiza) is a type of prostaglandin E1 analog that helps ease chronic constipation and IBS-C. It's especially helpful for those who haven't had success with fiber or osmotic laxatives.

Guanylate Cyclase-C Agonist

Linaclotide (Linzess) is another go-to option for IBS-C. It works locally in the gut to make stools softer and easier to pass.

How These Medications Work

- Lubiprostone increases fluid secretion in the small intestine by activating chloride channels, which boosts motility.
- Linaclotide stimulates intestinal cells to release chloride and bicarbonate into the lumen while reducing sodium absorption. The result? More water in the bowels and easier stools.

Who Benefits From These Drugs?

These medications are prescribed for:

- Chronic idiopathic constipation
- Opioid-induced constipation
- IBS-C in adults

They're especially helpful in reducing abdominal discomfort that often comes along with constipation.

What to Watch For

Common side effects include:

- Diarrhea
- Gas or bloating
- Stomach pain
- Abdominal distention
- No significant drug interactions have been reported.

Nursing Considerations

Assessment

- Evaluate bowel habits and GI history.
- Monitor for side effects and changes in stool pattern.
- Check fluid intake, dietary habits, and physical activity.
- Ensure the patient and family understand how the medication works.

Implementation

- Give on an empty stomach, at least 30 minutes before breakfast.
- Don't crush or chew enteric-coated tablets.
- Promote access to a toilet or bedpan.
- Encourage other healthy bowel habits—hydration, diet, and movement.

Evaluation

- The patient should experience more regular bowel movements.
- Abdominal pain should improve.
- The patient and caregivers should feel confident managing the medication.

Selective 5-HT3 Receptor Antagonist for IBS-D

Alosetron: Reserved for Tough Cases

Alosetron is prescribed for women with severe diarrhea-predominant IBS (IBS-D) who haven't responded to other treatments for at least 6 months.

Due to serious risks, this medication is only available through a restricted access program. Prescribers and patients must enroll.

How It Works

Alosetron blocks serotonin (5-HT3) receptors in the gut, which helps reduce abdominal pain, slow transit time in the colon, and decrease secretions—making it useful for IBS-D.

Who Shouldn't Take It

Avoid alosetron if the patient has:

- Constipation
- GI obstruction, stricture, or adhesions
- Toxic megacolon or GI perforation
- Ischemic colitis
- History of thrombophlebitis, Crohn's disease, ulcerative colitis, or diverticulitis

It hasn't been studied in pregnant or nursing women and may pose a higher risk of complications in older adults.

Serious Risks

- This medication has been linked to life-threatening side effects, including:
- Ischemic colitis (loss of blood flow to part of the colon)
- Severe constipation, leading to obstruction, toxic megacolon, or even perforation
- Stop the medication immediately if constipation develops.

Drug Interactions

Although data is limited, alosetron may:

- Interfere with metabolism of drugs like isoniazid, procainamide, and hydralazine
- Increase the risk of severe constipation when combined with other drugs that slow GI motility

Nursing Considerations

Assessment

- Take a thorough GI history before starting therapy.
- Watch closely for signs of constipation or complications.
- Monitor bowel movements and assess hydration status.

Implementation

- Time doses to avoid disruptions in daily routine.
- Ensure the patient understands the risks and requirements.
- Assist the patient in enrolling in the prescribing program and signing the necessary agreement.
- Educate on early signs of adverse effects and when to seek help.

Evaluation

- Patient should experience fewer IBS symptoms without serious complications
- Bowel patterns should stabilize.
- The patient and family should understand how to use the medication safely.

7.5. Obesity Medications: Tools to Support Health-Driven Weight Loss

Obesity medications aren't magic pills—but for people who are clinically obese, especially those with weight-related health conditions like diabetes, heart disease, or sleep apnea, these drugs can play a valuable role. They're not for cosmetic weight loss, but rather to support long-term health improvements when combined with a full weight management plan that includes diet, physical activity, and behavior change.

Types of Obesity Medications

There are several different types of drugs used to support weight loss, including:

- Appetite suppressants, like phentermine
- Fat blockers, like orlistat
- Serotonin receptor activators, like lorcaserin (Belviq)
- Newer agents, such as liraglutide (Saxenda) and Contrave (a combination of bupropion and naltrexone)

How They Work

Phentermine: This is a short-term appetite suppressant that boosts norepinephrine and dopamine levels in the brain, helping reduce hunger.

Lorcaserin: Targets specific serotonin (5-HT2C) receptors in the brain that help you feel full sooner. The exact mechanism is still being studied.

Orlistat: Works right in your gut. It blocks enzymes that break down fat, which prevents your body from absorbing about 30% of the fat you eat.

Liraglutide (Saxenda): This GLP-1 receptor agonist helps regulate blood sugar, slows stomach emptying, and suppresses appetite. It's not for people with type 2 diabetes, even though it's related to Victoza, a diabetes medication.

Contrave: Combines two medications—naltrexone (used to treat addiction) and bupropion (used for depression and smoking cessation)—to reduce cravings and emotional eating by working on the brain's reward and impulse-control centers.

What to Expect

These medications are generally prescribed for people with a BMI of 30 or higher, or 27 or higher if other health issues (like high blood pressure or diabetes) are also present.

Used properly and in combination with lifestyle changes, these drugs can:

- Help people lose weight

- Improve blood sugar and cholesterol
- Reduce the risk of serious health problems like stroke and heart attack

Side Effects to Know About

Phentermine: Can cause nervousness, dry mouth, constipation, and high blood pressure. It's not recommended for people with heart disease or a history of substance abuse.

Lorcaserin: May lead to headaches, low blood sugar, dry mouth, nausea, and fatigue.

Orlistat: Because it blocks fat absorption, it can cause gas with oily spotting, diarrhea, urgency, or fecal incontinence—especially if you eat a high-fat meal. These effects often lessen over time.

Liraglutide (Saxenda): May cause nausea, vomiting, diarrhea, and in rare cases, pancreatitis or thyroid tumors (warning labels apply).

Contrave: Can cause nausea, headache, insomnia, constipation, and increased heart rate. It's not for people with uncontrolled high blood pressure, seizure disorders, or those using opioids.

Important Drug Interactions

- Phentermine can increase risk of hypertension and anxiety, especially when taken with other stimulants or antidepressants.
- Combining orlistat with fat-soluble vitamins (A, D, E, K) may block their absorption—taking a multivitamin at least 2 hours apart is recommended.
- Using lorcaserin with other serotonergic drugs (like SSRIs or migraine meds) can cause serotonin syndrome—a potentially serious condition.

Nursing Care & Patient Support

Assessment

- Check for health risks related to obesity (heart disease, diabetes, sleep apnea).

- Monitor vital signs, weight, waist circumference, and BMI.
- Assess the patient's dietary habits, physical activity, and readiness to change.
- Review lab values, such as cholesterol, blood sugar, and blood pressure.

Key Nursing Diagnoses

- Imbalanced nutrition: More than body requirements
- Disturbed body image
- Deficient knowledge related to medication use

Planning Goals

- Patient will lower caloric intake and improve overall diet.
- Patient will achieve weight loss and improved self-image.
- Patient and family will understand how to take medications safely.

Implementation

- Emphasize that phentermine is for short-term use only.
- Avoid phentermine in patients with cardiovascular risk.
- Monitor blood pressure regularly.
- Ensure patients taking orlistat take a multivitamin daily, spaced 2 hours from the dose.
- Reinforce the importance of lifestyle changes—these medications are not a substitute for healthy habits.

Evaluation

- Patient experiences gradual and safe weight loss.
- Patient reports improved energy, health, and self-confidence.
- Patient and family show understanding of proper medication use and potential side effects.

7.6. Antiemetic Medications: Keeping Nausea in Check

Nausea and vomiting can be miserable. Whether it's caused by motion sickness, chemotherapy, surgery, or illness, antiemetic medications are designed to calm the stomach and reduce the urge to vomit—making a tough experience a little more manageable.

Types of Antiemetics

There are several types of antiemetics, each working a bit differently depending on the cause of the nausea:

- Antihistamines (like dimenhydrinate, diphenhydramine, meclizine) – helpful for motion sickness or nausea related to inner ear issues
- Phenothiazines (like prochlorperazine, promethazine) – used for moderate to severe nausea, including after surgery or during illness
- Serotonin (5-HT3) receptor antagonists (like ondansetron) – commonly used for chemo- or radiation-induced nausea and post-op care
- Cannabinoids (like dronabinol) – sometimes used for chemo-related nausea or when other medications haven't worked
- Neurokinin receptor antagonists (like aprepitant) – often used in combination with other antiemetics for severe chemotherapy nausea

Ondansetron is the most commonly used antiemetic in the U.S., known for being highly effective and well tolerated.

How They Work

Each type of antiemetic works in its own way to calm the body's nausea signals:

- Antihistamines block signals from the inner ear to the brain's vomiting center.

- Phenothiazines block dopamine in the brain's "chemoreceptor trigger zone," which is a fancy way of saying they interrupt the brain's nausea signals.
- 5-HT3 antagonists block serotonin both in the brain and gut—key pathways that trigger vomiting.
- Cannabinoids and neurokinin antagonists work through other central pathways to reduce severe nausea.

When They're Used

Antiemetics can help with:

- Motion sickness (best taken before symptoms begin)
- Postoperative nausea and vomiting
- Nausea from chemotherapy or radiation
- Severe illness-related vomiting (like from a virus or migraine)

Possible Drug Interactions

Antiemetics can interact with other medications, so it's important to use them carefully:

- Antihistamines and phenothiazines, when combined with other CNS depressants (like alcohol, opioids, or sleep aids), may increase drowsiness or confusion.
- These drugs can also cause anticholinergic effects—dry mouth, constipation, blurred vision, or difficulty urinating—especially when taken with similar medications.
- Some combinations can lead to rare but serious side effects like extrapyramidal symptoms (involuntary muscle movements).

Common Side Effects

- Drowsiness and dizziness are common, especially with antihistamines and phenothiazines.
- Dry mouth, blurry vision, or constipation may occur due to anticholinergic effects.

- Serotonin blockers may cause headache, fatigue, or mood changes.
- Phenothiazines may also cause low blood pressure, restlessness, or even fainting.

Everyone responds differently, so monitoring symptoms is key.

Nursing Process for Antiemetics

Assessment

- Check the patient's baseline symptoms, especially frequency and severity of nausea/vomiting.
- Evaluate for any potential drug interactions.
- Monitor fluid balance and hydration status.
- Assess the patient's understanding of the medication and its intended use.

Key Nursing Diagnoses

- Ineffective health maintenance due to nausea or underlying condition
- Risk for fluid volume deficit due to vomiting
- Deficient knowledge related to medication therapy

Planning Goals

- Patient will have reduced or no nausea/vomiting.
- Fluid balance will be maintained.
- Patient and caregivers will understand how and when to take the medication.

Implementation Tips

- Give antiemetics as prescribed—timing can make a big difference.
- For motion sickness, give 30–60 minutes before travel.
- Avoid subcutaneous injections—IM or oral forms are typically used.

- Inject IM medications into a large muscle, rotating sites if needed.
- Educate patients to avoid alcohol or driving until they know how the drug affects them.
- Remind them to stop antiemetics 4 days before allergy testing, as they can interfere with results.

Evaluation

- Nausea and vomiting are controlled.
- Patient remains well-hydrated with normal intake/output.
- Patient and family demonstrate confidence and knowledge in using the medication.

Chapter 8: Genitourinary Medicines

8.1. Medications That Support the Genitourinary System

The genitourinary (GU) system plays a big role in keeping your body balanced and functioning well. It's made up of two important parts:

- The urinary system, which includes your kidneys, ureters, bladder, and urethra
- The reproductive system, which includes the organs involved in sexual health and reproduction

Let's focus first on the urinary system, where the real behind-the-scenes work happens.

Why the Kidneys Deserve More Credit

Your kidneys do more than just make urine—they're powerhouses that help keep your whole body in check. Here's what they do:

- Filter your blood, removing waste and extra fluids as urine
- Balance electrolytes (like sodium, potassium, calcium) to keep nerves and muscles working properly
- Help regulate your body's pH, or acid-base balance
- Control blood pressure and blood volume by releasing an enzyme called renin
- Produce hormones and enzymes important for red blood cell production and blood vessel health
- Activate vitamin D, which helps your body absorb calcium

All of this work happens quietly every day—until something throws the system off balance. That's where medications can help.

Types of GU Medications

Several classes of medications are used to manage disorders in the genitourinary system. Each one supports a different function:

- Diuretics – Help your body get rid of extra fluid and sodium through urine. Often used for high blood pressure, heart failure, or swelling (edema).
- Urinary tract antispasmodics – Relieve bladder spasms and reduce symptoms like urgency, frequency, and leakage (especially helpful in overactive bladder).
- Erectile dysfunction (ED) drugs – Improve blood flow to help men with ED maintain an erection.
- Hormonal contraceptives – Used to prevent pregnancy by regulating hormones that control the menstrual cycle and ovulation.

The Big Picture

Whether the issue is high blood pressure, kidney stones, urinary urgency, or reproductive health, the right medications can support and protect your GU system. These drugs often work best when paired with healthy habits, like staying hydrated, eating well, and staying physically active.

8.2. Diuretics: Helping the Body Let Go of Extra Fluid

Diuretics—often called "water pills"—help your body get rid of extra fluid by encouraging your kidneys to flush out water and electrolytes (like sodium and potassium). These medications are a go-to option for conditions like high blood pressure, heart failure, kidney disease, and swelling (edema).

Thiazide and Thiazide-like Diuretics

These diuretics are mild to moderate in strength and often used for high blood pressure and swelling. They can also help prevent kidney stones and may surprisingly reduce urine output in diabetes insipidus—even though they're diuretics!

Common thiazide diuretics:

- Chlorothiazide (Diuril)
- Hydrochlorothiazide (HydroDIURIL, Microzide)

Thiazide-like options:

- Indapamide (Lozol)
- Chlorthalidone (Thalitone)
- Metolazone (Zaroxolyn)

How They Work

Thiazides prevent sodium from being reabsorbed in the kidneys—so it's flushed out in urine, dragging water along with it. They also lower blood pressure over time by helping relax small blood vessels. But they can deplete potassium and raise blood sugar, so labs need monitoring.

When Are They Used?

- High blood pressure (long-term control)
- Mild to moderate heart failure
- Swelling from kidney/liver issues
- Prevention of kidney stones

What to Watch For

- Low potassium (muscle cramps, weakness)
- Low sodium or dizziness
- High blood sugar
- Dehydration or frequent urination

If your patient has diabetes, kidney disease, or is on digoxin, monitor closely.

Nursing Tips

- Give early in the day to avoid nighttime bathroom trips

- Monitor daily weights (same time, same scale, same clothing)
- Watch electrolytes, especially potassium and sodium
- Encourage a potassium-rich diet or supplements if ordered
- Keep a urinal or bathroom easily accessible

Loop Diuretics: The Heavy Lifters

Loop diuretics like furosemide (Lasix), torsemide (Demadex), and ethacrynic acid (Edecrin) are your go-to meds when a stronger fluid removal is needed—like in severe heart failure, kidney disease, or massive swelling.

How They Work

Loop diuretics act in the "loop of Henle" (part of the kidney) to force the body to release a large amount of sodium and water. They also reduce blood pressure and increase blood flow to the kidneys and lungs.

Uses

- Severe heart failure
- Kidney failure
- Liver cirrhosis with fluid buildup
- Pulmonary edema
- High calcium levels (furosemide)
- Brain swelling (with mannitol)

Common Risks

- Dehydration and electrolyte imbalance (especially low potassium and sodium)
- Hearing issues with high doses (especially with ethacrynic acid)
- High blood sugar
- Uric acid buildup (watch for gout)

Nursing Care

- Monitor BP and heart rate, especially during rapid fluid shifts

- Watch for hypovolemia (low fluid volume) signs: dry mouth, low BP, dizziness
- Keep close tabs on weight, input/output, and labs (electrolytes, BUN, creatinine)
- Administer IV doses slowly to prevent a drop in BP
- Give early in the day to avoid nocturia
- Educate on using sunscreen due to possible photosensitivity

Key Nursing Diagnoses

- Risk for fluid volume depletion
- Risk for electrolyte imbalance
- Deficient knowledge about diuretic therapy

Evaluation Goals

- Patient maintains normal hydration and electrolyte levels
- Weight and swelling improve
- Patient and family can explain when and how to take the medication—and why it matters

Potassium-Sparing Diuretics: Holding On to Potassium While Flushing Out Fluid

Potassium-sparing diuretics are often used when there's a need to remove excess fluid without losing too much potassium. They don't have the powerful diuretic effects of other classes, but their ability to preserve potassium is their biggest benefit.

Common Examples:

- Spironolactone (Aldactone)
- Triamterene (Dyrenium)

How They Work

These medications act on the distal tubules and collecting ducts in the kidneys. They help get rid of sodium, water, calcium, and bicarbonate, but hold on to potassium and hydrogen ions—a big win for those at risk of low potassium.

Spironolactone goes a step further by blocking aldosterone, a hormone that usually tells the kidneys to retain sodium and water and dump potassium. By doing the opposite, spironolactone helps reduce fluid buildup and lowers blood pressure.

When They're Used

These drugs may be prescribed for:

- Swelling (edema)
- High blood pressure
- Heart failure
- Liver cirrhosis
- Hyperaldosteronism
- Hypokalemia caused by other diuretics

Spironolactone can also treat hirsutism (excess hair growth) in women with conditions like PCOS.

Drug Interactions

- Potassium supplements or ACE inhibitors increase the risk of hyperkalemia.
- Taking spironolactone with digoxin or lithium can raise toxicity risk.
- NSAIDs may weaken the diuretic effect.

Side Effects to Watch For

- High potassium levels (hyperkalemia)
- Gynecomastia (breast swelling in men)
- Menstrual irregularities in women
- Dizziness, headaches, vision changes

Nursing Care & Patient Tips

Assessment:

- Monitor blood pressure, pulse, and fluid status closely
- Watch for signs of hyperkalemia: muscle weakness, slow heart rate, or confusion
- Check lab values regularly (BUN, creatinine, electrolytes)
- Daily weights and input/output help track fluid shifts

Implementation:

- Give early in the day to avoid nighttime bathroom trips
- Avoid salt substitutes or potassium-rich foods unless prescribed
- Make sure patients know to rise slowly to avoid dizziness
- Keep urinals/bedpans close by for safety

Evaluation:

- Fluid and electrolyte levels stay within target range
- No adverse effects like dehydration or hyperkalemia
- Patient and family understand how and when to take the medication

Osmotic Diuretics: Pulling Fluid Where It Needs to Go

Osmotic diuretics are powerful medications used in urgent situations where fluid needs to shift quickly—like when there's brain swelling, high eye pressure, or acute kidney injury.

Examples:

- Mannitol (Osmitrol)
- Urea

How They Work

These drugs create an osmotic gradient—which basically means they pull water out of cells and into the bloodstream or into the kidneys to be excreted. This helps reduce pressure inside the skull or eyes and supports urine production in failing kidneys.

When They're Used

- Cerebral edema (swelling in the brain)
- Acute kidney failure
- High intraocular pressure
- Toxic substance elimination via the kidneys

Side Effects

- Fluid overload or electrolyte shifts
- Rebound increase in intracranial pressure (after initial drop)
- Headache, chest pain, tachycardia
- Rare but serious: seizures, thrombophlebitis, or pulmonary congestion

Nursing Care & Patient Tips

Assessment:

- Monitor vitals, urine output, and central venous pressure
- Watch closely for signs of circulatory overload (especially if urine output is low)
- Check neurological status and signs of increased ICP

Implementation:

- Administer slow IV infusion (over 3 minutes to hours, depending on reason)
- Use care to avoid IV infiltration, which can irritate or damage tissues
- Give in the morning to avoid sleep disruption
- Track weight and fluid balance daily
- Keep sodium and potassium labs on your radar

Evaluation:

- Fluid status remains stable

- Neurologic symptoms improve
- Patient and family understand the purpose of treatment and how to monitor for side effects

8.3. Urinary Tract Antispasmodics: Calming an Overactive Bladder

Urinary tract antispasmodics are medications designed to ease muscle spasms in the bladder and urinary tract. They help people struggling with an overactive bladder—a condition that can make daily life uncomfortable and unpredictable due to frequent urges, leaks, or difficulty holding urine.

Commonly Used Medications:

- Darifenacin (Enablex)
- Oxybutynin (Ditropan XL)
- Solifenacin (VESIcare)
- Tolterodine (Detrol)
- Trospium (Sanctura)

How They Work

These medications work by relaxing the bladder muscle. They block certain nerve signals—specifically, parasympathetic activity—that normally cause the bladder to contract. When this activity is reduced, the bladder muscle (called the detrusor muscle) relaxes, which helps reduce urgency, frequency, and incontinence episodes.

Oxybutynin also has anticholinergic effects, which is why dry mouth or constipation may occur.

How the Body Handles Them (Pharmacokinetics)

- Most of these drugs are taken orally and are absorbed quickly.
- Trospium, however, is poorly absorbed and is best taken on an empty stomach.
- All are processed by the liver and excreted through urine.
- They may cross the placenta and are also found in breast milk.

When They're Used

These medications are typically prescribed for people with:

- Overactive bladder
- Urge urinary incontinence
- Neurogenic bladder (in some cases, like with oxybutynin)

They're helpful for managing symptoms like sudden urges to urinate, frequent urination, and accidental leakage.

Drug Interactions

- Taking them with other anticholinergic drugs (like antihistamines or certain antidepressants) can intensify side effects like dry mouth or constipation.
- They may reduce the effect of phenothiazines (like Thorazine or Compazine) and haloperidol (Haldol).
- Trospium may interfere with how your body clears drugs like digoxin, metformin, or vancomycin, possibly increasing the levels of those medications in the blood.

Side Effects to Watch For

Some people may experience:

- Blurred vision
- Drowsiness or headaches
- Dry mouth or constipation
- Nausea or upset stomach
- Urinary retention
- Weight gain
- Angle-closure glaucoma (rare but serious—seek care if you notice vision changes)

Nursing Care & Patient Tips

Assessment:

- Check symptoms like urgency, frequency, and incontinence before starting treatment
- Use cystometry testing if ordered, to measure bladder function.
- Track intake and output to monitor effectiveness and fluid balance.

Key Nursing Diagnoses:

- Urge incontinence
- Low self-esteem due to incontinence
- Knowledge deficit about the medication

Goals:

- Patient has fewer incontinence episodes.
- Patient feels more confident and comfortable.
- Patient can take the medication correctly and safely.

Implementation Tips

- Follow dosage instructions carefully.
- Trospium should be taken on an empty stomach or 1 hour before meals.
- Offer small, frequent meals to help with nausea.
- Unless restricted, encourage plenty of fluids (2 to 3 liters/day) to help ease side effects like dry mouth or constipation.
- Help the patient understand that it may take time for full symptom relief.

Evaluation

- The patient reports relief from urgency and leakage.
- Fewer bathroom trips or accidents.
- Patient and family understand how the medication works and how to take it safely.

- Improved self-esteem and confidence in daily life.

8.4. Erectile Dysfunction Therapy: Supporting Confidence and Circulation

Erectile dysfunction (ED) happens when there's not enough blood flow to the penis to achieve or maintain an erection. This issue is often linked to vascular or nerve-related conditions. Fortunately, several medications can help by improving blood flow where it's needed most.

Common ED Medications:

- Sildenafil (Viagra)
- Tadalafil (Cialis)
- Vardenafil (Levitra)
- Alprostadil (Muse, Caverject, Edex)

How These Medications Work

- Sildenafil, tadalafil, and vardenafil all work by blocking the enzyme phosphodiesterase type 5 (PDE5). This boosts the natural levels of nitric oxide, a substance that helps relax smooth muscle in the penis and allows blood to flow in, leading to an erection.
- Alprostadil is a bit different. It's not taken by mouth—instead, it's injected directly into the penis or administered via a suppository. It works locally to increase blood flow by relaxing the smooth muscle in the erectile tissue.

What the Body Does With These Drugs

- Sildenafil, tadalafil, and vardenafil are well-absorbed when taken orally. They're processed by the liver and mostly excreted in feces.
- Alprostadil skips the GI tract altogether. It's metabolized in the lungs and then excreted through urine.

What They're Used For

- All of these medications are prescribed to treat erectile dysfunction.
- Sildenafil is also used for pulmonary arterial hypertension—a type of high blood pressure that affects the arteries in the lungs and heart.

Important Drug Interactions

- Avoid taking nitrates or alpha-blockers (like those used for chest pain or high blood pressure) with ED drugs. This combo can cause a dangerous drop in blood pressure.
- Drugs like ketoconazole, erythromycin, or ritonavir may raise the levels of ED medications in your system, increasing the risk of side effects.

Possible Side Effects

Mild to moderate effects can include:

- Headache
- Flushing (redness or warmth in the face)
- Indigestion
- Dizziness
- Changes in vision

Serious risks include:

- Cardiovascular events (heart attack, stroke, arrhythmias) especially in people with preexisting heart conditions
- Prolonged erection (lasting more than 4 hours), which can cause permanent damage
- Alprostadil may cause penile pain or bleeding at the injection site

Nursing Considerations and Patient Education

Assessment:

- Evaluate the patient's heart health before starting any ED medication.
- Monitor blood pressure, heart rate, and ECG, especially in those with known cardiovascular risks.
- Review the patient's medication list for potential interactions.

Nursing Diagnoses:

- Risk for decreased cardiac output due to drug-induced hypotension
- Risk for injury from prolonged erection (priapism)
- Deficient knowledge about proper medication use

Goals:

- Patient maintains stable heart function
- Patient understands proper use of ED medication
- No adverse complications from treatment

Implementation Tips

- Reinforce safety: ED meds do not protect against STIs or pregnancy.
- If using alprostadil: Show the patient how to use and inject it correctly. Stress the importance of aseptic technique and safe handling, as injection site bleeding can increase the risk of transmitting infections.
- Warn about timing: Patients taking HIV medications may experience enhanced effects, so it's critical to report side effects like dizziness or erections that last too long.
- Avoid alcohol and grapefruit juice while using these medications, as they may worsen side effects.

Evaluation

- Patient maintains healthy vital signs and cardiac output.

- No complications occur from prolonged erection or adverse reactions.
- Patient and family can clearly explain how and when to use the medication.

8.5. Hormonal Contraceptives: More Than Just Birth Control

Hormonal contraceptives are designed to prevent pregnancy by stopping ovulation and making it harder for sperm to meet an egg. They're available in several forms—pills, patches, rings, and intrauterine devices (IUDs)—and often contain a combination of estrogen and progestin hormones or progestin alone.

How They Work

Hormonal contraceptives work in a few key ways:

- Estrogen blocks the release of follicle-stimulating hormone (FSH), stopping the egg from maturing.
- Progestin prevents the release of luteinizing hormone (LH), which stops ovulation.
- Progestin also thickens cervical mucus, making it harder for sperm to reach the egg, and alters the lining of the uterus to prevent implantation.

Common Forms

- Combination Pills: Contain ethinyl estradiol (estrogen) with a progestin like desogestrel, norethindrone, or levonorgestrel.
- Progestin-Only Pills (Mini-pill): Used when estrogen isn't recommended.
- Patches: Applied to the skin, absorbed similarly to pills.
- Rings: A flexible silicone ring inserted into the vagina, releasing hormones over time.
- IUDs: Placed inside the uterus by a healthcare provider and release progestin slowly over months or years.

What They're Used For

- Primary use: Preventing pregnancy.
- Bonus benefit: The combination of ethinyl estradiol and norgestimate can also help treat moderate acne in young women under 15.

Potential Drug Interactions

Some medications and supplements can interfere with how hormonal contraceptives work. Watch out for:

- Antibiotics, seizure meds (like phenytoin, phenobarbital), and modafinil—they may lower effectiveness.
- Atorvastatin may increase estrogen levels.
- Prednisone can intensify the effects and side effects of birth control.
- Herbal supplements (especially St. John's wort) may reduce their effectiveness.
- Cyclosporine and theophylline may build up in the body and increase toxicity risk when taken with contraceptives.

Possible Side Effects

Hormonal contraceptives can cause a range of side effects, from mild to serious:

Common reactions include:

- Spotting between periods
- Nausea or upset stomach
- Breast tenderness
- Bloating
- Changes in weight or mood
- Acne or changes in skin
- Headaches
- Libido changes

Serious (but rare) reactions include:

- Blood clots (DVT, PE)
- Heart attack or stroke
- High blood pressure
- Liver issues or tumors

These risks are higher in smokers over age 35 or anyone with a history of blood clots or certain cancers.

Nursing Care & Patient Education

Assessment:

- Review the patient's medical history, especially for conditions like blood clots, high blood pressure, liver disease, breast cancer, or smoking.
- Monitor vital signs, especially blood pressure.
- Ask about migraine history, diabetes, or abnormal bleeding.
- Evaluate the patient's understanding of how to use her contraceptive method properly.

Common Nursing Diagnoses:

- Risk for ineffective protection due to incorrect use or drug interactions
- Risk for injury from side effects or complications
- Deficient knowledge about contraceptive use or safety

Teaching & Implementation

- Teach how to use contraceptives correctly—whether it's a pill, patch, or ring.
- Explain what to do if a dose is missed or if vomiting/diarrhea occurs.
- Stress that hormonal contraceptives do NOT protect against STIs. A barrier method like condoms is needed for STI protection.
- Review potential drug interactions and when to use a backup method (e.g., while taking antibiotics or seizure meds).

- Encourage patients to report unusual bleeding, severe headaches, leg pain, or shortness of breath, as these may signal serious complications.

Evaluation

- Patient remains pregnancy-free while on therapy.
- No signs of serious adverse reactions.
- Patient (and family, if applicable) demonstrates a clear understanding of how the contraceptive works, how to use it, and what to watch out for.

Chapter 9: Hematologic Medicines

9.1. Drugs That Work on the Blood (Hematologic System)

The hematologic system is essentially your body's blood and all the parts that help it do its job. This includes:

- Plasma — the liquid that carries cells, nutrients, hormones, and waste
- Red blood cells (RBCs) — carry oxygen throughout the body
- White blood cells (WBCs) — fight infection
- Platelets — help your blood clot when you're bleeding

When something goes wrong with any of these components, medications can step in to help. Here are the main types of drugs used to treat blood-related conditions:

1. Hematinic Drugs

These are typically iron, vitamin B12, or folic acid supplements. They help boost red blood cell production—especially important in cases of anemia or nutritional deficiencies.

2. Anticoagulants (Blood Thinners)

These drugs don't actually thin the blood, but they help prevent clots from forming or growing. They're often prescribed for people at risk for strokes, heart attacks, deep vein thrombosis (DVT), or pulmonary embolism.

3. Thrombolytics (Clot Busters)

Thrombolytic drugs are used in emergency situations to break up dangerous blood clots—like those that cause strokes or heart attacks. They work fast and are typically given in hospital settings.

9.2. Hematinic Drugs – Giving Blood a Boost

When it comes to making healthy red blood cells (RBCs), your body needs the right building blocks. Hematinic drugs help by supplying those essentials—like iron, vitamin B12, and folic acid—so your body can make more hemoglobin, the protein that carries oxygen in your blood. These medications are typically used to treat various forms of anemia.

Iron Supplements: Fueling Red Blood Cell Production

Iron supplements are the most common way to treat iron deficiency anemia—the kind that happens when your body doesn't have enough iron to make hemoglobin.

Common forms include:

- Ferrous sulfate
- Ferrous gluconate
- Ferrous fumarate
- Iron dextran (injection)
- Iron sucrose (injection
- Sodium ferric gluconate complex (injection)

How It Works in the Body

Iron is mainly absorbed in the small intestine (specifically, the duodenum and jejunum). Your body absorbs more when iron stores are low or RBC production ramps up. But if you already have enough iron, absorption drops significantly.

Once absorbed, iron travels through the bloodstream bound to a protein called transferrin. It's stored in the liver, spleen, and bone marrow, and used mostly to make hemoglobin. Any excess is excreted in sweat, urine, stool—and even breast milk.

Who Needs It

- People with iron deficiency anemia
- Children between 6 months and 2 years (a period of rapid growth)
- Pregnant women (to support fetal development)
- Patients with bowel disorders or undergoing dialysis (who may need injectable forms)

Tips & Cautions

- Iron works better when taken on an empty stomach, but it can cause stomach upset. Vitamin C (like orange juice) can help with absorption.
- Avoid taking iron with foods or meds that block absorption—like dairy, tea, coffee, and antacids.
- Liquid iron can stain teeth, and the supplements can darken stools (that's normal!).

Side Effects

- Upset stomach
- Constipation
- Stained teeth (from liquid iron)
- Rarely, allergic reactions with injections

Vitamin B12: Essential for Nerve Health and Cell Growth

Vitamin B12 (cyanocobalamin or hydroxocobalamin) is crucial for forming RBCs and maintaining healthy nerve function. It's used to treat pernicious anemia, which happens when your body can't absorb enough B12 due to lack of a substance called intrinsic factor.

How It Works

B12 is absorbed in the small intestine—but only with help from intrinsic factor, which is made in the stomach. If your body doesn't produce this, you'll need high-dose oral B12 or injections.

Once absorbed, B12 is stored in the liver and slowly released as your body needs it.

Who Needs It

- People with pernicious anemia
- Those who've had gastric surgery or bowel disorders
- Patients with nutritional deficiencies (e.g., vegetarians, elderly)

Side Effects

- Usually well-tolerated
- Rarely, hypersensitivity reactions like rash or anaphylaxis with injections

Folic Acid: Key for Red Blood Cell Formation (and a Healthy Pregnancy!)

Folic acid is a type of B vitamin your body uses to make new cells—including RBCs. It's especially important during periods of rapid growth, like infancy, adolescence, and pregnancy.

Who Needs It

- People with folic acid deficiency anemia (often seen in alcoholics, elderly, or people with intestinal disorders)
- Pregnant women (to prevent neural tube defects)
- People on medications that lower folic acid levels (like methotrexate or anticonvulsants)

How It Works

- Folic acid is absorbed in the small intestine and stored throughout the body. It helps cells divide and grow—especially blood cells.

Side Effects

- Rare, but may include rash, nausea, irritability, or trouble sleeping
- In large doses, it can reduce the effectiveness of certain seizure medications

Nursing Considerations (for all hematinics)

Assessment:

- Check for signs of deficiency (fatigue, pallor, lab values like hemoglobin and hematocrit)
- Monitor response to therapy

Implementation:

- Give oral iron with water or juice—not milk
- Use the Z-track method for iron injections to avoid skin staining
- Encourage foods rich in iron and folic acid (leafy greens, meats, legumes)

Evaluation:

- Look for improvement in lab values and symptoms
- Ensure the patient and family understand the purpose and side effects of therapy

Epoetin Alfa & Darbepoetin Alfa: Helping the Body Make Red Blood Cells

When your body isn't making enough red blood cells—especially due to kidney problems—medications like epoetin alfa and darbepoetin alfa can step in and help. These drugs mimic a natural hormone called erythropoietin, which is normally produced by the kidneys in response to low oxygen levels. Their job? Stimulating the bone marrow to produce more red blood cells (RBCs).

How They Work in the Body

- Epoetin alfa and darbepoetin alfa are given either subcutaneously (under the skin) or through an IV.
- After injection, epoetin alfa peaks in 5–24 hours, while darbepoetin alfa takes a bit longer—up to 72 hours.
- Their effects last several days, which means you don't need to take them daily.
- Both are cleared by the kidneys, so dosing may be adjusted in patients with kidney issues.

What They're Used For

These drugs are prescribed for people with normocytic anemia, a condition where your RBCs are normal in size but low in number. Common situations include:

- Chronic kidney disease (CKD) – when the kidneys can't make enough natural erythropoietin
- HIV treatment-related anemia – especially if taking zidovudine
- Before major surgery – to reduce the need for blood transfusions

Potential Side Effects

While these drugs are incredibly helpful, they're not without risks. Common side effects include:

- High blood pressure (most common)
- Headache
- Joint or muscle pain
- Nausea or vomiting
- Swelling (edema)
- Fatigue or dizziness
- Diarrhea

- Skin reactions at the injection site

More serious but less common risks include:

- Seizures
- Blood clots (deep vein thrombosis, stroke, or heart attack)
- Chest pai
- Tumor growth in cancer patients
- Pure red cell aplasia (a rare bone marrow condition)

Things Nurses Watch For

Assessment:

- Check iron levels first—these meds don't work well without enough iron!
- Monitor hemoglobin, hematocrit, and reticulocyte count to track progress.
- Watch for changes in blood pressure—especially in the early stages.
- Be alert for side effects, especially cardiovascular ones.

Common Nursing Diagnoses:

- Ineffective health maintenance due to underlying anemia
- Risk for injury from low RBCs or side effects
- Deficient knowledge about how to manage therapy at home

Helpful Nursing Tips

- Give IV doses slowly as directed.
- Patients on dialysis may also need heparin to prevent clotting.
- Encourage iron-rich foods and monitor nutritional intake.
- Offer comfort care for symptoms like nausea or fatigue.
- Be sure the patient and family understand how the medication works and why iron intake is important.

How We Know It's Working

- Blood counts return to a healthy range.

- Symptoms of anemia (like fatigue and weakness) improve.
- Patient and family feel confident managing the therapy and understand the risks.

9.3. Anticoagulant Drugs: Keeping Clots in Check

Anticoagulants are medications that slow down the blood's ability to clot, helping to prevent dangerous clots that can cause heart attacks, strokes, or deep vein thrombosis (DVT). These drugs don't dissolve clots that already exist—but they can stop them from getting bigger and prevent new ones from forming.

Let's break down the different types:

- Heparin and low-molecular-weight heparins (like enoxaparin)
- Oral anticoagulants (like warfarin)
- Antiplatelet drugs (like aspirin and clopidogrel)
- Direct thrombin inhibitors
- Factor Xa inhibitors

Heparin and Heparin Derivatives

Heparin is a fast-acting anticoagulant often used in hospitals. It works by boosting a natural protein in your body called antithrombin III, which blocks the clotting process. It doesn't affect clotting factors already made by the liver, so it can't break up clots, only prevent new ones.

Low-molecular-weight heparins (like enoxaparin and dalteparin) are easier to use because they're given by injection under the skin and require less monitoring than traditional heparin.

How Heparin Works in the Body

- Given through IV or subcutaneously—not by mouth or IM (too risky).
- Starts working fast when given IV, but less predictable through injection.

- Broken down by the liver and leaves the body through urine.

It blocks clotting factors like Xa and thrombin, depending on the dose. Low doses are used to prevent clots, while higher doses treat active clotting issues.

When Is Heparin Used?

Doctors use heparin to:

- Treat and prevent DVT and pulmonary embolism
- Manage atrial fibrillation, where blood can pool in the heart
- Help during surgery or dialysis, where blood circulates outside the body
- Support patients recovering from a heart attack

Important Drug Interactions

Heparin interacts with a lot of drugs, so providers keep a close watch. It may increase bleeding risk if taken with:

- NSAIDs like ibuprofen
- Antiplatelets like aspirin or clopidogrel
- Iron injections

Protamine sulfate is the antidote in case of serious bleeding.

Side Effects to Watch For

Heparin is generally safe when monitored carefully, but possible side effects include:

- Bleeding (most common, and treatable)
- Bruising or skin reactions
- Low platelet count (thrombocytopenia)

Nursing Care with Heparin

- Monitor PTT (a blood test) to make sure clotting time is in the safe zone.
- Watch for signs of bleeding—gums, urine, stool, or bruising.

- Avoid IM injections if possible.
- Keep protamine sulfate nearby for emergencies.
- Educate the patient and family on safety precautions.

Oral Anticoagulants: Warfarin (Coumadin)

Warfarin is the go-to oral anticoagulant in the U.S. It takes a few days to kick in because it works by blocking vitamin K, which your liver needs to make clotting factors.

Given by mouth

- Absorbed quickly, but doesn't start working for 36–48 hours
- Broken down in the liver, and drug interactions are very common

When Is Warfarin Used?

- Doctors prescribe warfarin to:
- Prevent and treat DVT
- Reduce stroke risk in people with atrial fibrillation
- Support patients with mechanical heart valves
- Prevent clots after surgery

Watch Out for Interactions

Warfarin is tricky. Many drugs and even certain foods can either increase bleeding risk or make the drug less effective. Key culprits include:

- Vitamin K-rich foods (like spinach or kale)
- Alcohol
- NSAIDs and antibiotics
- Other blood thinners

Antidote alert: Vitamin K or fresh frozen plasma can reverse its effects in case of bleeding.

Common Side Effects

- Bleeding (especially GI bleeding)
- Easy bruising
- Birth defects—warfarin is not safe during pregnancy

Nursing Considerations for Warfarin

- Monitor PT and INR blood levels regularly
- Teach the patient to stick to a consistent diet (especially with vitamin K)
- Keep vitamin K on hand in case of serious bleeding
- Use bleeding precautions (soft toothbrush, no contact sports, etc.)

Antiplatelet Drugs: Keeping Arteries Clear

These drugs prevent platelets from clumping together and forming clots, especially in arteries. They're commonly used to prevent:

- Heart attacks
- Strokes
- Clotting in patients with stents or heart disease

Examples include:

- Aspirin
- Clopidogrel
- Dipyridamole
- Ticlopidine

For more severe cases, IV antiplatelet drugs like abciximab or eptifibatide are used in the hospital.

How They Work

Each drug works slightly differently:

- Aspirin blocks an enzyme needed to activate platelets.
- Clopidogrel and ticlopidine interfere with platelet binding.

- Dipyridamole increases levels of a platelet-blocking chemical.
- IV drugs block a key receptor (glycoprotein IIb/IIIa) on the surface of platelets.

Antiplatelet Drugs: Keeping Arteries Clear

Some blood clots form in arteries when platelets stick together and build up. Antiplatelet medications help prevent that. They're especially useful for people at risk of heart attacks, strokes, or blood clots from stents or artificial heart valves.

When They're Used

- Aspirin is the go-to drug for people who've had a heart attack or unstable angina, and for men at risk of transient ischemic attacks (TIAs)—brief reductions in brain blood flow.
- Clopidogrel is used to lower the chance of stroke or heart-related death in people who've had a recent heart attack or stroke, or have peripheral artery disease. It's also used during procedures like angioplasty or bypass surgery.
- Dipyridamole is usually paired with a coumarin drug after heart valve surgery to prevent clotting.
- Ticlopidine is used to prevent strokes in people who can't take aspirin—but due to serious side effects, it's used only when absolutely necessary.
- Eptifibatide, tirofiban, and abciximab are IV medications used during emergencies or heart procedures like angioplasty.

Drug Interactions to Watch Out For

Combining antiplatelet drugs with others that affect blood clotting can increase the risk of bleeding. For example:

- NSAIDs, heparin, and oral anticoagulants make bleeding more likely.
- Aspirin can raise levels of methotrexate and valproic acid, making toxicity more likely.
- Antacids can lower the effectiveness of ticlopidine.

239

- Some drugs like cimetidine can increase the risk of bleeding with ticlopidine.

Heads up: Don't mix ticlopidine with heparin, warfarin, or aspirin unless specifically directed—it hasn't been well studied and could be dangerous.

Common Side Effects

- Aspirin may cause stomach pain, heartburn, nausea, and even some blood in the stool.
- Clopidogrel can cause headaches, joint pain, flu-like symptoms, and rarely a serious condition called thrombotic thrombocytopenic purpura (TTP).
- Ticlopidine might bring on nausea, diarrhea, rashes, or even a drop in white blood cells (neutropenia).
- Dipyridamole can lead to dizziness, flushing, and mild stomach upset.
- IV drugs like abciximab and tirofiban mostly increase the risk of bleeding.

Nursing Considerations

- Monitor closely for signs of bleeding (gums, urine, stool).
- Keep an eye on vital signs, blood counts, and salicylate levels if on long-term aspirin.
- Avoid unnecessary needle sticks to reduce the chance of bruising or hematoma.
- Always give aspirin with food or milk to protect the stomach.
- Stop antiplatelet meds 5–7 days before surgery, unless otherwise directed.

Direct Thrombin Inhibitors: A Newer Way to Thin the Blood

These drugs, like dabigatran, argatroban, and bivalirudin, block thrombin, a key enzyme in clot formation.

How They Work

They prevent clots by:

- Blocking thrombin so it can't convert fibrinogen into fibrin, which forms the structure of a blood clot.
- Stopping platelet activation and aggregation.
- Working on both free-floating and clot-bound thrombin (something heparin can't do).

When They're Used

- Dabigatran is taken by mouth to prevent strokes in people with non-valvular atrial fibrillation.
- Argatroban is used for patients who've developed heparin-induced thrombocytopenia (HIT) and might be undergoing procedures like angioplasty.
- Bivalirudin is used for people with unstable angina going through PTCA (angioplasty), usually with aspirin.

Important: Don't use bivalirudin in people with active bleeding, recent brain surgery, or serious kidney disease without adjusting the dose.

Drug Interactions & Cautions

- Avoid using these drugs with other anticoagulants or thrombolytics unless specifically directed.
- Be cautious with patients who are bleeding, have recent surgery, or have liver or kidney disease.
- Dabigatran should be stored in its original bottle—not in pill organizers—as it's sensitive to moisture and heat.

Side Effects

- Bleeding is the main concern—especially for patients at high risk.

Other issues can include:

- Nausea, vomiting, abdominal cramps

- Headache
- Injection site bruising
- Rare cases of intracranial bleeding or retroperitoneal hemorrhage

Nursing Care

- Monitor labs (PT, PTT, INR), blood pressure, and vital signs.
- Check for bleeding in stool, urine, or vomit.
- Educate patients on signs of bleeding and when to call the provider.
- Use infusion pumps for IV forms, and avoid unnecessary injections to prevent bruising.

Factor Xa Inhibitors: Another Step Forward

Fondaparinux is the only FDA-approved Factor Xa inhibitor in the U.S. It's used to prevent DVTs and pulmonary embolism, especially after hip or knee surgery.

How It Works

It boosts the activity of antithrombin III, which then blocks factor Xa—a key player in the clotting cascade. This interruption helps stop thrombus (clot) formation.

Pharmacokinetics

- Given subcutaneously, fondaparinux is absorbed quickly.
- Peaks within 2 hours, and its effects last 17–24 hours.
- Leaves the body mainly through urine.

Watch for Interactions & Side Effects

Don't give with other bleeding-risk medications unless advised.

Possible side effects:

- Bleeding
- Nausea or constipation

- Rash
- Anemia
- Swelling

Nursing Tips

- Inject only into fatty tissue, and rotate sites.
- Don't mix with other meds in the same syringe.
- Watch for signs of bleeding, and always double-check labs (PT, INR, PTT, CBC).
- Keep the patient and family informed about why the drug is needed and how to stay safe during treatment.

9.4. Thrombolytic Drugs: Busting Clots When Time Is Critical

Thrombolytic drugs—sometimes called "clot busters"—are powerful medications used to dissolve dangerous blood clots in emergencies like heart attacks, strokes, or pulmonary embolism. These medications work fast and are typically given through an IV line or directly into the blocked blood vessel.

Commonly used thrombolytics include:

- Alteplase (tPA)
- Reteplase
- Tenecteplase

How They Work

These drugs work by converting plasminogen (a natural substance in your blood) into plasmin, which then breaks down fibrin—the main protein that holds a blood clot together. Think of plasmin as the body's natural clot dissolver, and thrombolytics as the key that unlocks it.

How They Move Through the Body

Once given:

- They enter the bloodstream immediately and begin working right away.
- They're cleared quickly by the liver, so their effects don't last long.
- They do not cross the placenta, so they're not likely to reach a developing fetus.

When They're Used

Thrombolytics are life-saving when used in time. They're most effective within 6 hours of the start of symptoms. They're used to treat:

- Acute myocardial infarction (heart attack)
- Acute ischemic stroke
- Pulmonary embolism (clot in the lungs)
- Peripheral arterial occlusion (blocked blood flow to limbs)
- Blocked dialysis or IV catheters

Specific uses:

- Alteplase: for heart attacks, strokes, PEs, and blocked IV lines.
- Reteplase and Tenecteplase: mainly for treating heart attacks.

Drug Interactions to Know

- Combining thrombolytics with heparin, anticoagulants, antiplatelet drugs, or NSAIDs can significantly increase the risk of bleeding.
- Aminocaproic acid can reverse the effects of some thrombolytics if bleeding becomes a problem.

Side Effects

The most serious risk is bleeding, both at visible sites and internally. Allergic reactions can also happen—especially with older agents like streptokinase.

Nursing Considerations

Assessment

- Review the patient's medical history and reason for thrombolytic therapy.
- Monitor closely for signs of bleeding, especially in urine, stool, or vomit.
- Regularly check vital signs, lab results (PT, INR, PTT, CBC), and cardiac rhythm.
- Watch for changes in cardiopulmonary status, such as breathing difficulty or chest pain.

Nursing Diagnoses

- Risk for decreased tissue perfusion due to clot
- Risk for fluid volume deficit due to bleeding
- Knowledge deficit related to treatment

Planning Goals

- Improved circulation and oxygen delivery to tissues
- Stable fluid levels and vital signs
- Clear understanding of treatment by the patient and family

Implementation

- Follow facility protocols closely when preparing and giving these medications.
- Use an infusion pump to ensure safe, controlled delivery.
- Avoid unnecessary injections or blood draws, which can cause bruising or bleeding.
- Keep antiarrhythmic medications on hand, as clots breaking up can sometimes cause rhythm issues.
- Use bleeding precautions, and avoid invasive procedures while the drug is active.
- Administer heparin alongside thrombolytics if ordered, following guidelines carefully.

Evaluation

- Patient shows improved circulation and oxygen delivery, as seen in vital signs and overall condition.
- No signs of internal or external bleeding are present.
- Patient and family understand the purpose, risks, and expectations of the treatment.

Chapter 10: Endocrine Medicines

10.1. Understanding Drugs That Affect the Endocrine System

The endocrine system is made up of glands and organs found throughout the body. What makes it special is that it produces and releases hormones—the body's chemical messengers. These hormones travel through the bloodstream to reach specific organs or tissues, where they trigger a response.

Hormones play a vital role in keeping things balanced, helping the body respond to stress, regulate metabolism, control growth and development, manage blood sugar, and even control reproduction. The body releases these hormones as needed, based on internal cues and feedback signals.

A System of Checks and Balances

The endocrine system works closely with the central nervous system to keep the body in a state of homeostasis, or internal balance. It's like your body's built-in thermostat—constantly adjusting levels to maintain stability.

When the Balance is Off: Medications Step In

Sometimes, the body doesn't produce enough hormones—or produces too much. In those cases, medications can help restore that balance. These drugs are used to treat hormone imbalances or endocrine-related disorders, and they fall into a few main categories:

- Natural hormones and their synthetic versions, like insulin for diabetes or glucagon for low blood sugar.
- Hormonelike substances, which mimic the body's own hormones.

- Drugs that stimulate or suppress hormone production, helping to either boost a needed response or calm an overactive one.

10.2. Medications for Diabetes and Blood Sugar Management

When it comes to managing diabetes, it's all about keeping blood sugar levels in a safe, healthy range. The body uses insulin—a hormone made in the pancreas—to help regulate those levels. People with diabetes either don't make enough insulin or can't use it effectively.

To help with that, we use two key types of medications:

- Hypoglycemic drugs: These lower blood sugar levels. They include insulin and oral antidiabetic medications.
- Hyperglycemic drugs: These raise blood sugar levels when they drop too low. Glucagon is the main one in this category.

Why Blood Sugar Goes Out of Balance

Diabetes mellitus is a long-term condition that causes the body to either not produce insulin (Type 1 diabetes) or not use it properly (Type 2 diabetes). This leads to elevated blood sugar levels and affects how the body processes carbohydrates, fats, and proteins.

Blood sugar can drop too low if:

- A patient takes too much medication,
- Skips meals or doesn't eat enough,
- Or exercises more than usual without adjusting food or meds.

Insulin: The Lifesaving Hormone

Type 1 diabetes always requires insulin, and many people with Type 2 may eventually need it—especially during illness, stress, or surgery.

Types of Insulin

Insulin types are categorized by how fast they act:

- Rapid-acting: lispro (Humalog)

- Short-acting: regular insulin (Humulin R)
- Intermediate-acting: NPH
- Long-acting: glargine (Lantus), detemir (Levemir)

How Insulin Works in the Body

- It helps store sugar as glycogen in the liver.
- It promotes protein and fat building.
- It slows the breakdown of stored nutrients.
- It balances fluid and electrolytes.
- It also helps move potassium into cells, which is useful when treating high potassium levels.

When Is Insulin Prescribed?

- For Type 1 diabetes
- For Type 2 diabetes when oral medications aren't enough
- During stressful events like surgery or infection
- For pregnant women who can't take oral meds
- To treat complications like DKA (diabetic ketoacidosis) or HHNK syndrome
- For hyperkalemia (too much potassium), even in people without diabetes

Possible Side Effects of Insulin

- Low blood sugar (hypoglycemia) is the most common concern.
- Reactions like lipodystrophy (fat tissue changes), allergic responses, or insulin resistance can also occur.

What Nurses Monitor

- Blood sugar levels, regularly and especially before meals or meds
- Ketones in urine if sugar levels are high
- Injection sites for signs of irritation
- Hemoglobin A1C to monitor long-term glucose control

Tips for Giving Insulin

- Store it properly and check expiration dates.
- Mix cloudy insulin by gently rolling the vial—never shake it.
- Use the correct syringe and injection technique.
- Rotate injection sites to avoid skin problems.
- Be ready to treat low blood sugar with glucose tablets, juice, or glucagon if needed.

Oral Antidiabetic Drugs: Helping the Pancreas (and Beyond)

These are used mainly for Type 2 diabetes when diet and exercise alone aren't enough. They work in different ways, depending on the drug type:

Types and Actions

- Sulfonylureas (e.g., glipizide, glyburide): Stimulate the pancreas to release more insulin.
- Biguanides (e.g., metformin): Reduce sugar production in the liver and improve insulin sensitivity.
- Thiazolidinediones (e.g., pioglitazone): Help cells use insulin better.
- Alpha-glucosidase inhibitors (e.g., acarbose, miglitol): Slow sugar absorption from food.
- Meglitinides (e.g., repaglinide): Help the pancreas produce insulin around mealtimes.
- Incretin-based therapies (e.g., sitagliptin): Help maintain post-meal insulin response.

How Nurses Help with Oral Antidiabetic Therapy

- Monitor blood sugar and kidney/liver function.
- Watch for low blood sugar, especially if combining meds.
- Teach patients to take meds as prescribed and follow a healthy eating plan.

- Reinforce the importance of regular activity and follow-up appointments.

Combining Oral Antidiabetics with Insulin

Sometimes, a single treatment approach just isn't enough. For people who don't get the results they need from insulin or oral antidiabetic medications alone, combining the two might be the answer. It's a strategy that helps many patients reach better glucose control.

Drug Interactions: A Balancing Act

When oral antidiabetic drugs interact with other medications, the most common risks are low blood sugar (hypoglycemia) or high blood sugar (hyperglycemia).

What Can Cause Blood Sugar to Drop Too Low

Hypoglycemia is more likely to happen when certain oral antidiabetics—especially sulfonylureas or metformin—are combined with:

- Alcohol
- Steroids (anabolic)
- Certain antibiotics (chloramphenicol, sulfonamides)
- Fluconazole
- MAO inhibitors
- Cimetidine
- Warfarin
- Ranitidine

Metformin has a lower risk of causing hypoglycemia when used alone.

What Can Push Blood Sugar Too High

Drugs that may reduce the effects of oral antidiabetics (leading to hyperglycemia) include:

- Corticosteroids
- Rifampin

- Sympathomimetics (like decongestants)
- Thiazide diuretics

Important note: If a patient is having a procedure that requires IV contrast dye, metformin should be paused beforehand—there's a risk of acute kidney injury.

Side Effects to Watch Out For

Sulfonylureas may cause:

- Nausea or stomach fullness
- Low sodium levels
- Rash or sun sensitivity
- Blood abnormalities
- Water retention

Metformin may lead to:

- Metallic taste
- Nausea or vomiting
- Abdominal discomfort

Acarbose can cause:

- Gas
- Diarrhea
- Abdominal pain

Thiazolidinediones may lead to:

- Weight gain
- Swelling

How Nurses and Providers Support Patients

Assessment

- Monitor blood sugar regularly—especially for those switching from insulin to oral meds.
- Watch for side effects or signs of poor drug response.

- Evaluate how well the patient is following the treatment plan.
- Gauge the patient's (and their family's) understanding of how the medication works.

Common Nursing Diagnoses

- Ineffective health maintenance due to unfamiliarity with diabetes care
- Risk for injury due to hypoglycemia
- Deficient knowledge about diabetes medication

Planning Goals

- Maintain stable blood sugar levels
- Minimize the risk of complications or injury
- Help patients and families feel confident about managing the medication

Nursing Actions and Education

- Be aware that micronized glyburide isn't the same as regular glyburide—it may require dose adjustments.

Timing matters:

- Sulfonylureas: Take 30 minutes before meals.
- Metformin: Take with morning and evening meals.
- Acarbose or miglitol: Take with the first bite of each main meal.
- Liver monitoring: For patients on thiazolidinediones, check liver function regularly.
- Most patients take oral antidiabetics once daily, but twice-daily dosing may work better for higher doses.
- Always treat low blood sugar quickly—give fast-acting glucose if the patient can swallow, or glucagon/IV glucose if not.

Reminders:

- Insulin may be needed temporarily during stress, illness, or surgery.

- Encourage a balanced diet and exercise plan.
- Teach patients how to spot and respond to high or low blood sugar.

Glucagon: A Life-Saver for Severe Lows

Glucagon is a hormone the body naturally makes to raise blood sugar. When used as a medication, it's most often given during emergencies—like severe hypoglycemia (low blood sugar) when the person is unresponsive or can't eat or drink.

How Glucagon Works

- Fast-acting: Works within minutes after subcutaneous (subcut), intramuscular (IM), or IV injection.
- Main site of action: The liver, where it helps release stored glucose.
- Broken down by the liver and kidneys and removed from the body fairly quickly.

When It's Used

- Emergencies: Severe hypoglycemia when oral glucose isn't an option.
- Radiology: Sometimes used to slow down the GI tract during imaging.

Drug Interactions and Side Effects

- The main interaction is with oral anticoagulants, which may increase the risk of bleeding.
- Side effects are rare, but nausea and vomiting can occur.

How Nurses Manage Glucagon Therapy

Assessment

- Check blood sugar levels regularly—especially in times of stress or illness.
- Watch for any reactions or interaction with other medications.

- Make sure the patient stays hydrated if they're vomiting.
- Teach patients and families when and how to use glucagon.

Nursing Diagnoses

- Risk for injury due to hypoglycemia
- Deficient knowledge about managing low blood sugar

Goals

- Maintain stable blood sugar levels
- Prevent injury during hypoglycemic episodes
- Ensure families know what to do in an emergency

Implementation Tips

- Reconstitute glucagon as instructed before injection.
- After giving it, try to wake the patient quickly and give a snack with carbohydrates once they're alert.
- If the patient doesn't respond, be ready to give IV dextrose.
- Always notify the prescriber if glucagon is used.
- Monitor for rebound hypoglycemia, and watch for vomiting.

What Success Looks Like

- Blood glucose returns to safe levels
- The patient avoids injury or complications
- The family feels confident managing emergencies

10.3. Thyroid & Antithyroid Medications: Finding the Right Balance

The thyroid gland may be small, but it plays a big role in how your body works. When it's not making enough hormone, we call that hypothyroidism. When it's working overtime and producing too much, that's hyperthyroidism. Thankfully, we have medications that can help restore balance in both cases.

Thyroid Hormone Replacement (For Hypothyroidism)

When your thyroid is underactive, you may need a boost from thyroid medications. These drugs replace the hormones your thyroid isn't making enough of.

Types of Thyroid Hormone Medications:

Natural (from animal sources):

- Desiccated thyroid (Thyroid USP): contains both T3 and T4
- Thyroglobulin: also contains T3 and T4

Synthetic (lab-made versions):

- Levothyroxine (T4) – most commonly prescribed
- Liothyronine (T3)
- Liotrix (T3 and T4 combo)

How They Work in Your Body:

Thyroid medications help:

- Boost metabolism
- Regulate heart rate and energy
- Improve how your body uses proteins, carbs, and fats
- Increase kidney blood flow and help with fluid balance

They also can help treat:

- Various forms of hypothyroidism
- Goiter prevention (enlarged thyroid)
- Thyroid cancer (as part of treatment or suppression)

What to Watch For:

If the dosage is too high, it can speed up your body too much, leading to:

- Palpitations or fast heartbeat
- Anxiety or nervousness
- Weight loss, diarrhea

- Trouble sleeping
- Irregular periods

Important Drug Interactions:

- Warfarin: Can increase bleeding risk.
- Cholestyramine/Colestipol: Reduce absorption.
- Digoxin: Thyroid drugs can lower digoxin levels.
- Antiseizure drugs (phenytoin, carbamazepine) and rifampin: May make thyroid meds less effective.

Nursing Care Tips for Thyroid Replacement:

Assessment

- Monitor thyroid labs (TSH, T3, T4).
- Watch for signs of under- or over-treatment.
- Check blood pressure and heart rate.
- Monitor response to anticoagulants if the patient is on one.

Implementation

- Start with low doses and adjust slowly.
- Give the medication at the same time daily, ideally in the morning before food.
- Don't stop the drug suddenly—this is usually a lifelong treatment.
- Make sure patients know to expect it to take several weeks before they feel better.

Antithyroid Medications (For Hyperthyroidism)

When your thyroid is in overdrive, antithyroid medications help slow it down. These drugs are most often used in conditions like Graves' disease.

Common Antithyroid Medications:

Thioamides (block hormone production):

- Propylthiouracil (PTU): works quickly, used in more severe cases or in pregnancy (first trimester)
- Methimazole: preferred for long-term treatment; taken once daily

Iodides (short-term control and surgery prep):

- Stable iodine (Lugol's solution)
- Radioactive iodine: destroys overactive thyroid tissue

How They Work:

- PTU and Methimazole stop the thyroid from making hormones.
- Stable iodine prevents the release of hormones.
- Radioactive iodine damages the thyroid over time to reduce its activity.

Important Things to Know:

- PTU is safer during early pregnancy; methimazole is used later.
- It can take several weeks before these meds start working fully.
- Radioactive iodine is often a one-time treatment, but takes weeks or months to take effect.
- Surgery may be needed in some cases.

Side Effects:

PTU and methimazole can cause low white blood cell counts, increasing infection risk.

Iodine solutions may cause:

- Metallic taste
- Swollen salivary glands
- Mouth/throat irritation

Rare but serious side effect: agranulocytosis (dangerously low white blood cells)

Nursing Care Tips for Antithyroid Therapy:

Assessment

- Check thyroid levels regularly.
- Monitor white blood cell counts (to catch agranulocytosis early).
- Watch for signs of hypothyroidism as the medication takes effect.

Implementation

- PTU is usually taken several times a day; methimazole is taken once daily.
- Use juice to mask the taste of iodine drops.
- Patients should be taught to report fever, sore throat, or unusual tiredness immediately.

How We Know It's Working:

For thyroid replacement:

- Energy levels improve
- Weight stabilizes
- Lab results normalize

For antithyroid therapy:

- Heart rate slows
- Anxiety and heat intolerance improve
- Goiter shrinks
- Thyroid hormone levels stabilize

10.4. Pituitary drugs

Pituitary drugs either replace or help regulate the hormones that the pituitary gland normally makes. These medications are split into two groups:

- Anterior pituitary drugs: Help regulate growth, development, thyroid, adrenal, and reproductive function.
- Posterior pituitary drugs: Help with fluid balance and uterine muscle contractions.

Anterior Pituitary Drugs: Helping Hormones Do Their Job

These drugs are often used when the body needs a little help regulating its natural hormone rhythms.

Types of Anterior Pituitary Medications

- Adrenocorticotropics (corticotropin, cosyntropin): Help assess or treat adrenal gland function.
- Growth hormones (somatrem, somatropin): Stimulate growth, especially in children with growth hormone deficiency.
- Gonadotropins (chorionic gonadotropin, menotropins): Aid fertility in both men and women.
- Thyrotropics (thyrotropin alfa, protirelin): Used in thyroid cancer care or to test thyroid function.

How They Work

These drugs act as chemical messengers, telling other glands to start or stop hormone production. They're not taken by mouth because your digestive system would break them down—most are given by injection.

Why They're Prescribed

- To stimulate growth in children with growth hormone deficiency.
- To test adrenal or thyroid function.
- To help with fertility.
- To treat conditions like multiple sclerosis, thyroid cancer, or hormonal imbalances.

Things to Watch Out For

Drug Interactions

- These medications can interact with:
- Vaccines, NSAIDs, diuretics, or barbiturates
- Certain antiseizure drugs may reduce their effectiveness.
- Some drugs like estrogens or lithium can increase or alter hormone levels.

Side Effects

- Hypersensitivity reactions (rash, swelling, breathing issues)
- Cushing's syndrome from long-term use of corticotropin (too much cortisol)
- Changes in blood sugar, weight, or blood pressure

Nursing Tips and Patient Care

Assessment

- Check for changes in growth (for kids).
- Monitor hormone levels, vital signs, and weight.
- Look for signs of hormone imbalance or allergic reactions.
- Ask about the patient's understanding of their treatment.

Implementation

- Follow dosing instructions carefully—some need to be given at specific times or with food.
- Use the correct injection techniques, and rotate injection sites if needed.
- Store medications properly (some require refrigeration).

Education

- Teach patients and families about the purpose of the medication, possible side effects, and when to seek help.
- Explain that some therapies are short-term (like diagnostic tests), while others may be lifelong.

Posterior Pituitary Drugs: Managing Fluids and Labor

These drugs come into play when the body needs help holding onto fluids or regulating uterine contractions.

Common Posterior Pituitary Medications

- ADH (antidiuretic hormone): Desmopressin, Vasopressin
- Oxytocin: Stimulates labor and postpartum healing

What They Treat

- Neurogenic diabetes insipidus (causes excessive urination)
- Low blood pressure in critical care
- Postpartum bleeding
- Inducing or reinforcing labor
- Helping the uterus contract after childbirth

Important Safety Info

Interactions

- Alcohol and lithium may reduce the effect of ADH.
- Certain anesthetics can increase side effects or cause complications when used with oxytocin.
- Oxytocin, when used with vasopressors, can raise blood pressure significantly.

Adverse Reactions

- For ADH: Risk of water retention, low sodium, headaches, seizures
- For oxytocin: Risk of overly strong contractions, water intoxication, or postpartum bleeding

Nursing Considerations for Posterior Pituitary Therapy

Assessment

- Monitor fluid balance: daily weights, urine output, and blood pressure
- Watch for signs of water intoxication (confusion, headache, drowsiness)
- Monitor uterine contractions and fetal heart rate if giving oxytocin

Implementation

- ADH: Adjust dose based on fluid loss; teach proper use of nasal spray or injection.
- Oxytocin: Only give by IV infusion, not IV push. Keep magnesium sulfate nearby to stop contractions if needed.
- Stop the infusion if contractions are too frequent or too strong and call the provider.

How You Know It's Working

- For ADH: Normal urine output and stable sodium levels
- For Oxytocin: Labor progresses safely or postpartum bleeding stops
- Patients report feeling better and understand their treatment plan

10.5. Understanding Estrogen Therapy

Estrogens are hormones that play a big role in the female body—helping regulate everything from menstrual cycles to reproductive health. When the body doesn't produce enough estrogen on its own, medication can step in to restore balance.

What Are Estrogens Used For?

Estrogen medications—either natural or synthetic—are commonly prescribed for:

- Relieving menopause symptoms (like hot flashes or vaginal dryness)
- Replacing hormones in women with low estrogen due to early menopause, surgery, or certain medical conditions
- Supporting hormone levels in women with primary ovarian failure or hypogonadism
- Palliative treatment for some types of breast cancer in postmenopausal women and for prostate cancer in men

Types of Estrogen Medications

There are two main kinds:

- Natural estrogens: like estradiol or estropipate
- Synthetic estrogens: such as ethinyl estradiol or estradiol valerate

These are available in different forms—pills, patches, creams, injections, and vaginal rings or suppositories—depending on what works best for the patient's needs and preferences.

How It Works in the Body

Estrogen medications act on tissues like the breasts, uterus, and urinary tract to help restore hormone balance. They help promote protein and DNA production, which supports tissue health and overall function.

How They're Processed

Once taken, estrogens are well absorbed and travel through the bloodstream. They're broken down in the liver and mostly leave the body through the kidneys.

What to Watch For: Interactions and Side Effects

Drug Interactions

Some medications can change how estrogen works in your body:

- May decrease effectiveness: Certain antibiotics, anti-seizure meds (like phenytoin), and rifampin

- May increase clot risk: Anticoagulants like warfarin may be less effective
- Estrogens can also interfere with folic acid absorption, which might lead to deficiency

Possible Side Effects

Most people do well on estrogen, but it can occasionally cause:

- High blood pressure
- Blood clots (which can lead to DVT, stroke, or heart attack)
- Vaginal bleeding
- Breast tenderness or swelling
- Changes in weight or mood

Nursing Care and Patient Guidance

Assessment

- Take a full health history before starting therapy
- Check vital signs and perform a physical exam, including breast and pelvic exams

For long-term use, monitor:

- Blood pressure
- Liver function
- Cholesterol and lipid levels
- Weight changes
- Glucose levels (especially in diabetics)

Ongoing Monitoring

- Watch for signs of clot formation (leg pain/swelling, chest pain, sudden headaches)
- If the patient is also on blood thinners (like warfarin), monitor clotting labs (PT/INR)
- Educate the patient about potential side effects and when to call the doctor

Medication Administration Tips

- Follow prescribed schedules: Often given in cycles (e.g., 3 weeks on, 1 week off)
- Application instructions: Show patients how to apply topical forms or insert vaginal forms correctly
- Know when to pause: Stop estrogen therapy if blood clots are suspected and call the provider immediately

Educating the Patient

- Make sure the patient understands:
- Why they're taking estrogen
- How to take it safely
- What signs to watch for (like chest pain, vision changes, or leg swelling)
- That hormone therapy is usually short-term and should be reevaluated regularly

Goals of Therapy

- The patient's symptoms improve (for example, less hot flashes or more regular cycles)
- The patient avoids serious complications like clots or hypertension
- The patient and their family feel confident in managing the medication and understanding its purpose

Chapter 11: Psychotropic Medicines

11.1. Medications for Mental Health Conditions

In this chapter, we'll explore medications that help manage different mental health conditions, including anxiety, depression, attention deficit hyperactivity disorder (ADHD), psychotic disorders, and sleep-related issues. The goal is to understand how these drugs work and their role in helping people lead healthier, more balanced lives.

11.2. Sedative and Hypnotic Medications

Sedatives are medications that help calm the mind, ease tension, or reduce excitement, often causing drowsiness. At higher doses, they become hypnotics, promoting a state similar to natural sleep. There are three primary types of these drugs:

- Benzodiazepines
- Barbiturates
- Nonbenzodiazepine-nonbarbiturate medications

Benzodiazepines: Calming the Mind

Benzodiazepines have a range of uses beyond just sedation. They're commonly known as "chill pills" for their calming effects. Popular benzodiazepines for sedation include alprazolam, estazolam, flurazepam, lorazepam, temazepam, and triazolam.

How Benzodiazepines Work (Pharmacokinetics)

Benzodiazepines are quickly absorbed into your body, entering your bloodstream efficiently and traveling swiftly to your brain. How fast they take effect depends on their absorption rate, with flurazepam and triazolam working especially quickly. The drug's distribution in your body affects how long the sedative effects last. For instance, triazolam spreads widely but leaves your system quickly.

Typically, benzodiazepines are taken orally, but in emergencies, they may be given through injection. Your liver processes them, and they leave your body mainly through urine.

How Benzodiazepines Affect the Brain (Pharmacodynamics)

Benzodiazepines work by activating specific receptors (GABA) in the brain's reticular activating system (RAS), which manages alertness and wakefulness. Higher doses cause deeper sedation by suppressing activity in this area.

Unlike some other sleep medications, benzodiazepines generally don't reduce the quality of REM sleep (deep sleep with rapid eye movements), making them preferable to barbiturates.

When Benzodiazepines are Used (Pharmacotherapeutics)

Doctors prescribe benzodiazepines to:

- Help patients relax before surgery
- Treat insomnia and anxiety
- Provide sedation during anesthesia
- Manage alcohol withdrawal symptoms
- Control seizures
- Relax muscles

Important Drug Interactions

Combining benzodiazepines with other central nervous system depressants like alcohol or certain medications can dangerously amplify sedation, causing decreased alertness, impaired coordination, breathing difficulties, and even death. Additionally, drugs like hormonal contraceptives or antifungal medications may increase benzodiazepine levels, heightening the risk of side effects or toxicity.

Possible Side Effects

Common side effects include:

- Memory loss
- Fatigue
- Muscle weakness
- Dry mouth
- Nausea, vomiting
- Dizziness and balance issues

Benzodiazepines can also cause lingering drowsiness, impaired daytime functioning, or rebound insomnia. They carry risks of dependence and withdrawal.

Special Consideration for Seniors

Elderly individuals should use benzodiazepines cautiously because these medications may accumulate, increasing risks for side effects. Doctors typically recommend lower doses that are slowly adjusted upward if needed.

Barbiturates: Powerful Sedation

Barbiturates significantly reduce central nervous system activity. Common examples include phenobarbital and secobarbital.

How Barbiturates Work

Barbiturates reduce brain activity at lower doses, leading to drowsiness. Higher doses can dangerously suppress breathing and brain functions.

Barbiturate Uses

They're commonly used for:

- Short-term daytime sedation
- Insomnia relief
- Preoperative sedation
- Anxiety relief

- Seizure control

However, barbiturates carry higher risks of tolerance, dependence, and overdose compared to benzodiazepines, which are generally safer and preferred today.

Drug Interactions and Risks

Barbiturates interact with numerous drugs, potentially decreasing their effectiveness or increasing toxic effects. Particularly dangerous are interactions with other CNS depressants, which can cause profound sedation or respiratory depression.

Side Effects of Barbiturates

Common adverse effects include:

- Excessive sleepiness
- Headaches
- Depression
- Slow heart rate, low blood pressure
- Breathing difficulties
- Dizziness, nausea, vomiting, stomach pain

Nursing Considerations for Sedatives and Hypnotics

When caring for patients on these medications, healthcare providers should:

- Regularly assess anxiety levels, sleep patterns, and overall well-being.
- Monitor vital signs and possible side effects.
- Educate patients and families about the medications, safe use, and risks.
- Implement safety measures to prevent falls or injuries due to sedation.
- Avoid abrupt discontinuation to prevent withdrawal symptoms or worsening conditions.

Nonbenzodiazepine-Nonbarbiturate Sleep Medications

Nonbenzodiazepine-nonbarbiturate medications are commonly prescribed as short-term sleep aids to help people experiencing simple insomnia. They include medications like:

- Eszopiclone
- Zaleplon
- Zolpidem

Temporary Sleep Helpers

These medications are intended only for short-term use. It's important to collaborate with your healthcare provider to discover healthier, long-lasting strategies for better sleep.

How the Body Handles Them (Pharmacokinetics)

Nonbenzodiazepine-nonbarbiturate sleep aids are quickly absorbed from the stomach and intestines. They're metabolized (broken down) by the liver and removed from your body through urine.

How They Work (Pharmacodynamics)

Scientists aren't exactly sure how these drugs work, but they seem to have calming effects similar to barbiturates, slowing down activity in the brain to help you fall asleep.

Common Uses (Pharmacotherapeutics)

Healthcare providers typically use these medications for:

- Short-term relief from insomnia
- Sedation before surgical procedures
- Relaxation before EEG (brainwave) tests

Drug Interactions

Combining these medications with other central nervous system (CNS) depressants, like alcohol or certain pain medications, can enhance drowsiness and slow breathing significantly, potentially causing extreme sedation, coma, or even death.

Possible Side Effects

The most common side effects of these drugs are related to dosage and may include:

- Nausea or vomiting
- Upset stomach
- Residual drowsiness or "hangover effect" (which can sometimes lead to breathing difficulties or even respiratory failure)

Nursing Care for Patients

For patients prescribed these medications, nurses typically follow these steps:

Assessment

- Understand and evaluate the patient's underlying health condition.
- Regularly check if the medication is effectively improving the patient's sleep.
- Monitor for side effects or interactions with other medications.
- Evaluate the patient's and family's understanding of the medication and its use.

Key Nursing Diagnoses

- Insomnia related to the patient's underlying health conditions
- Risk of injury due to potential drowsiness and sedation
- Lack of understanding about the prescribed medication

Goals of Care

- Improved sleep quality for the patient
- Ensuring the patient remains safe and injury-free
- Patient and caregivers clearly understand medication use, precautions, and potential risks

Implementation (Practical Steps)

- Give the medication exactly as prescribed and closely watch for its effects.
- If using liquid forms, dilute to minimize unpleasant taste.
- Administer just before bedtime for maximum effectiveness.
- Store suppositories in a refrigerator to maintain effectiveness.
- Avoid long-term use, as the effectiveness decreases after approximately two weeks and dependence may develop. Suddenly stopping these medications after prolonged use may trigger withdrawal symptoms.
- Advise the patient to avoid tasks needing alertness or coordination. If hospitalized, provide supervision and safety measures (especially important for elderly patients).
- Encourage the patient to immediately inform their healthcare provider of side effects like excessive sedation or hangover feelings, allowing dosage adjustments if necessary.

Evaluation (Checking Outcomes)

- The patient reports improved sleep with medication use.
- The patient stays safe without any injury or harm from sedation effects.
- Both patient and caregivers demonstrate a clear understanding of how to safely use the medication.

11.3. Medications for Anxiety (Antianxiety Drugs)

Antianxiety medications, often called anxiolytics, are among the most frequently prescribed drugs in the United States. They primarily help manage anxiety disorders, offering relief to people struggling with overwhelming worry or fear. The three main categories include:

- Benzodiazepines
- Barbiturates
- Buspirone

Benzodiazepines: Familiar Faces for Anxiety Relief

While benzodiazepines and barbiturates were mentioned earlier as sedatives and sleep aids, they're also widely used to treat anxiety.

Common benzodiazepines specifically used for anxiety include:

- Alprazolam
- Chlordiazepoxide
- Clonazepam
- Clorazepate
- Diazepam
- Lorazepam
- Oxazepam

At lower doses, benzodiazepines soothe anxiety by acting on areas of the brain that regulate emotions, particularly the limbic system. This allows people to feel calmer without significant drowsiness.

Buspirone: A Different Approach to Anxiety

Buspirone belongs to its own unique class called azaspirodecanedione derivatives, setting it apart from benzodiazepines and barbiturates.

Advantages of buspirone include:

- Less sedation, so it doesn't make you feel overly sleepy
- Doesn't enhance the sedative effects of alcohol or other calming medications
- Lower potential for addiction or misuse

How Buspirone Works in the Body (Pharmacokinetics)

Buspirone is quickly absorbed, processed extensively by the liver, and produces at least one active byproduct before exiting the body through urine and feces.

Buspirone's Effects in the Brain (Pharmacodynamics)

The precise workings of buspirone are still somewhat unclear. However, it doesn't interact with GABA receptors like benzodiazepines do. Instead, it appears to influence serotonin receptors, acting on areas of the midbrain associated with anxiety regulation.

When Buspirone is Effective (Pharmacotherapeutics)

Buspirone is particularly useful in managing generalized anxiety disorder, especially in people who have not previously used benzodiazepines. However, it's not suitable when immediate anxiety relief is necessary because it takes longer to become effective (usually 1-2 weeks).

Buspirone is not recommended for ordinary daily stress, despite its low risk of addiction and absence of significant abuse potential.

Potential Drug Interactions

Unlike other anxiety medications, buspirone doesn't dangerously interact with alcohol or sedatives. However, mixing buspirone with certain antidepressants known as MAO inhibitors may cause severe increases in blood pressure.

Common Side Effects

- Patients might experience:
- Dizziness
- Lightheadedness
- Insomnia (difficulty sleeping)
- Rapid heartbeat or palpitations
- Headache

Nursing Care for Patients on Buspirone

Nurses caring for patients using buspirone typically follow these guidelines:

Assessment

- Evaluate the patient's anxiety levels before and regularly during therapy.
- Watch closely for side effects and possible drug interactions.
- Ensure the patient and family understand the medication and its use.

Key Nursing Diagnoses

- Anxiety due to the patient's underlying condition
- Fatigue caused by medication side effects
- Lack of understanding about medication use

Goals for Patient Care

- Reduced anxiety symptoms
- Minimal fatigue or side effects
- Patient and caregivers fully understand medication guidelines

Practical Nursing Interventions

- If switching from benzodiazepines, avoid abrupt discontinuation to prevent withdrawal symptoms.
- Administer the medication with food or milk to minimize stomach discomfort.
- Adjust the dose as recommended by the healthcare provider.
- Caution patients about driving or engaging in activities that require full mental alertness until they know how the medication affects them.
- Inform patients that improvement usually begins within 7-10 days, but full effectiveness may take up to 3-4 weeks.

Evaluating Patient Outcomes

- Patient experiences significant anxiety relief.
- Patient reports reduced fatigue and side effects.
- Patient and family demonstrate a clear understanding of medication use and safety.

11.4. Antidepressants and Mood Stabilizers

Antidepressant and mood stabilizing medications help manage mood disorders—conditions that affect how you feel, causing prolonged sadness (depression) or periods of heightened excitement (mania).

Treating Depression (Unipolar Disorders)

Depression, characterized by persistent feelings of sadness or loss of interest, is typically treated with:

- Selective serotonin reuptake inhibitors (SSRIs)
- Monoamine oxidase inhibitors (MAOIs)
- Tricyclic antidepressants (TCAs)
- Other antidepressants

Treating Bipolar Disorder

Bipolar disorder involves mood swings between depression and mania (extreme excitement or irritability). Lithium is commonly prescribed to stabilize these mood shifts.

SSRIs: Safer Options for Depression

SSRIs, designed to have fewer side effects than older antidepressants, are among the most frequently prescribed antidepressants today. Common SSRIs include:

- Citalopram
- Escitalopram
- Fluoxetine
- Fluvoxamine
- Paroxetine
- Sertraline

How SSRIs Work

SSRIs increase serotonin levels in the brain by blocking its reabsorption, helping regulate mood and emotions.

Uses Beyond Depression

SSRIs also effectively treat anxiety, panic disorders, eating disorders, and some personality or impulse control disorders. Always follow specific medication instructions for approved uses.

Possible Drug Interactions

Combining SSRIs with certain drugs, especially MAOIs, can cause severe and even life-threatening reactions. Always inform healthcare providers about all medications you're taking.

Side Effects to Watch For

Common side effects include anxiety, trouble sleeping, fatigue, changes in heartbeat, sexual dysfunction, and skin rashes. Suddenly stopping SSRIs can lead to withdrawal symptoms.

Important Safety Note: SSRIs have a warning regarding increased risk of suicidal thoughts, especially in younger patients. Close monitoring is essential.

Nursing Care with SSRIs

- Regularly assess mood and side effects.
- Provide medications in the morning to avoid sleep disturbances.
- Adjust doses carefully for elderly patients or those with liver or kidney conditions.

MAO Inhibitors: Powerful but Cautious Choices

MAO inhibitors, such as phenelzine and tranylcypromine, are strong antidepressants especially helpful for patients who haven't responded to other treatments.

How MAOIs Work

MAOIs prevent the breakdown of certain mood-regulating neurotransmitters, increasing their availability and easing depressive symptoms.

Conditions Treated by MAOIs

Effective in managing depression, panic disorders, eating disorders, post-traumatic stress disorder, and certain chronic pain conditions.

Dietary and Drug Precautions

MAOIs interact dangerously with specific medications and foods high in tyramine (e.g., aged cheese, red wine, processed meats), causing severe hypertension. Careful dietary monitoring is essential.

Side Effects of MAOIs

Common reactions include dizziness, low blood pressure upon standing, headaches, restlessness, insomnia, gastrointestinal issues, and dry mouth. Serious reactions require immediate medical attention.

Nursing Care with MAOIs

- Closely monitor vital signs, mood changes, and dietary habits.
- Educate patients about dietary restrictions and possible interactions.
- Plan carefully with healthcare providers when surgery is needed.
- Be prepared to manage hypertensive emergencies.

Evaluating Treatment Success

For both SSRIs and MAOIs, effective treatment is shown through improved mood, reduced depressive symptoms, patient safety, and clear patient and family understanding of medication guidelines and precautions.

TCAs: Older but Effective Options

TCAs are an older class of antidepressants that are still used today, especially when newer drugs don't work well. They help manage depression, especially when it creeps in slowly and comes with symptoms like insomnia, weight loss, or lack of appetite.

Some common TCAs include:

- Amitriptyline
- Nortriptyline
- Imipramine
- Doxepin
- Desipramine
- Clomipramine
- Protriptyline
- Trimipramine
- Amoxapine

How They Work

TCAs help lift mood by boosting the levels of norepinephrine and serotonin in the brain—two neurotransmitters involved in mood regulation. They also block other receptors (like for histamine and acetylcholine), which can cause side effects like drowsiness or dry mouth.

What They're Used For

Besides depression, TCAs can help with:

- Migraine prevention
- Panic disorder
- Obsessive-compulsive disorder (OCD)
- Bed-wetting (enuresis) in children
- Diabetic nerve pain
- ADHD (in some cases)

They can also be paired with mood stabilizers in bipolar depression.

Important Safety Notes

- Start low, go slow. It can take 1 to 4 weeks to feel the full benefit.

- Watch for side effects, including drowsiness, dizziness, low blood pressure, dry mouth, and in rare cases, heart rhythm problems or blood disorders.
- Never stop suddenly—you should taper down gradually to avoid withdrawal-like symptoms.
- Desipramine carries a black box warning about an increased risk of suicidal thinking in children, teens, and young adults.

Drug Interactions

TCAs can react with many other drugs:

- Can raise blood pressure when combined with certain stimulants
- May worsen side effects when taken with MAO inhibitors or anticholinergics
- Can lower the effectiveness of blood pressure meds like clonidine

Nursing Tips

- Monitor mood changes, vital signs, and for signs of overdose or suicidal thoughts.
- Watch for dry mouth, urinary retention, or constipation—dose adjustments may be needed.
- Check EKGs for patients over 40 or with heart conditions.

Other Antidepressants You Might See

There are other antidepressants outside the TCA and SSRI classes that work in unique ways:

Examples include:

- Bupropion (Wellbutrin) – may also help with smoking cessation
- Venlafaxine & Duloxetine – called SNRIs, they affect serotonin and norepinephrine
- Trazodone – often used at night to help with sleep

How They Help

These medications also work by tweaking brain chemicals to stabilize mood. They're often chosen when people don't respond well to SSRIs or TCAs, or when they have specific symptoms like poor sleep or anxiety.

Side Effects to Watch For

- Bupropion – may cause anxiety, tremors, or increase seizure risk (especially at high doses)
- SNRIs – can cause dizziness, nausea, or sleepiness
- Trazodone – often causes drowsiness and lightheadedness

Lithium: A Mood Stabilizer

Lithium is one of the oldest and most effective treatments for bipolar disorder, especially for controlling manic episodes and preventing mood swings.

How It Works

Lithium helps calm the brain by reducing the release of norepinephrine and possibly boosting serotonin uptake. The exact way it works is still being researched.

Why Monitoring Is Critical

Lithium has a narrow therapeutic range, meaning there's a small window between an effective dose and a toxic one. Too much lithium can lead to:

- Tremors
- Confusion
- Slurred speech
- Seizures

You'll need regular blood tests to monitor lithium levels, kidney and thyroid function, especially early in treatment or after dose changes.

Common Side Effects

- Thirst and frequent urination
- Upset stomach or metallic taste
- Slight hand tremors

Red Flags

Call your healthcare provider if you notice:

- Severe fatigue
- Worsening mood
- Unusual confusion
- Vision changes

Drug and Food Interactions

- NSAIDs and diuretics can raise lithium levels dangerously
- Low sodium diets can also increase toxicity risk, while high sodium intake can reduce lithium's effectiveness

Tips for Safe Use

- Take with food and drink plenty of water
- Never skip blood tests
- Avoid abrupt changes in diet (especially salt)
- Watch for dehydration (hot days, vomiting, or diarrhea can raise lithium levels)

11.5. Antipsychotic Medications: What You Need to Know

Antipsychotic drugs are powerful medications used to help manage psychosis, including symptoms like hallucinations, delusions, disorganized thinking, and severe mood disturbances—most commonly associated with conditions like schizophrenia, bipolar disorder, and mania.

What Are They Called?

These drugs go by different names depending on who you're talking to:

- Antipsychotics – because they treat psychotic symptoms.
- Major tranquilizers – because they calm agitation.
- Neuroleptics – because they can sometimes cause movement-related side effects.

Two Main Categories

Antipsychotic drugs fall into two main types:

1. Atypical Antipsychotics (Newer)

These are considered first-line treatments for schizophrenia and are often better tolerated with fewer movement-related side effects.

Common examples:

- Aripiprazole (Abilify)
- Olanzapine (Zyprexa)
- Quetiapine (Seroquel)
- Risperidone (Risperdal)
- Ziprasidone (Geodon)
- Lurasidone (Latuda)
- Clozapine (Clozaril)
- Brexpiprazole (Rexulti)

How Atypical Antipsychotics Work

They block dopamine receptors (which helps reduce psychosis), but not as strongly as older drugs. They also block serotonin receptors, which may help with mood symptoms and reduce the risk of severe side effects like muscle stiffness and tremors.

What They Treat

- Schizophrenia (both positive symptoms like hallucinations and negative symptoms like flat affect)
- Bipolar disorder (manic or mixed episodes)
- Depression (when other treatments don't work)

- Some behavioral symptoms in autism or dementia

Side Effects to Watch For

- Weight gain (especially with olanzapine and clozapine)
- Sedation (more common with quetiapine and aripiprazole)
- Heart rhythm issues (ziprasidone is not advised for people with heart conditions)
- Movement disorders (risperidone at higher doses)
- Agranulocytosis – a serious blood condition linked with clozapine

Drug Interactions

These medications can interact with a wide range of drugs, including:

- Blood pressure meds (can cause low BP)
- Other sedatives or alcohol (can intensify drowsiness)
- Drugs affecting liver enzymes (P450 system) which can raise or lower levels of antipsychotics
- Smoking – can reduce the effectiveness of some medications like olanzapine

Nursing Considerations

- Watch for movement changes or tardive dyskinesia (involuntary twitching or facial movements)
- Monitor for signs of sedation, weight gain, or blood disorders
- Don't stop the medication suddenly
- Teach patients to avoid alcohol and to report symptoms like sore throat, fever, or confusion

Typical Antipsychotics (Older Medications)

These are the original antipsychotic medications and are still used, though less often due to higher risk of movement disorders.

Common drugs include:

- Haloperidol (Haldol)

- Fluphenazine
- Chlorpromazine
- Thioridazine
- Thiothixene

How They Work

Typical antipsychotics block dopamine receptors more aggressively, which makes them effective for treating psychosis but also increases the risk of extrapyramidal symptoms (EPS), like:

- Muscle rigidity
- Restlessness
- Tremors
- Tardive dyskinesia

Side Effects and Safety

- EPS (including neuroleptic malignant syndrome, a rare but life-threatening reaction)
- Sedation, dry mouth, blurred vision
- Constipation or urinary retention
- Drop in blood pressure (especially after injections)
- Long-term use can lead to irreversible movement disorders

Monitoring & Labs

- Get baseline labs before starting: ECG, liver and kidney tests, electrolytes
- Monitor for mood changes, weight gain, and EPS every 6 months or more often if needed
- If giving chlorpromazine, monitor bilirubin levels weekly for the first month

Tips for Nurses and Caregivers

- Never stop abruptly unless there's a medical emergency
- Store and prepare medications according to instructions

- Reassure patients and families that medication takes time to work, sometimes several weeks
- Provide emotional support as patients adjust to treatment
- Encourage regular follow-up and lab monitoring

11.6. Stimulants: Getting Focused

Stimulants are a class of psychotropic medications commonly prescribed to treat Attention-Deficit/Hyperactivity Disorder (ADHD). They help manage symptoms like inattention, impulsivity, and hyperactivity, making it easier for patients—especially children and teens—to focus, stay on task, and perform better in school or work.

Common Stimulants

Some of the most commonly prescribed stimulant medications include:

- Dextroamphetamine
- Methylphenidate (Ritalin, Concerta)
- Mixed amphetamine salts (like Adderall)

How They Work (Pharmacodynamics)

Stimulants work by boosting the activity of dopamine and norepinephrine—two key brain chemicals involved in attention, motivation, and emotional regulation. They do this by:

- Blocking reuptake (so the brain keeps using these neurotransmitters longer)
- Releasing more from storage sites
- Inhibiting the enzyme (MAO) that breaks them down

The result? Better focus, calmer behavior, and more organized thinking.

How the Body Processes Them (Pharmacokinetics)

- Stimulants are well-absorbed when taken by mouth.
- Methylphenidate has a significant first-pass effect—meaning the liver breaks down a good portion of it before it enters the bloodstream.

- These drugs are processed mainly in the liver and excreted in the urine.

What They're Used For (Pharmacotherapeutics)

- ADHD: They're the first-line treatment for both children and adults.
- Narcolepsy: Dextroamphetamine and methylphenidate can help reduce sudden sleep attacks and improve wakefulness.

Drug Interactions to Be Aware Of

- Avoid using stimulants within 14 days of stopping an MAO inhibitor, as this can lead to dangerous side effects.

Methylphenidate may:

- Lower the effectiveness of guanethidine (a BP medication)
- Enhance the effects of TCAs, warfarin, and some seizure medications

Possible Side Effects

Dextroamphetamine

- Restlessness, tremors
- Trouble sleeping
- Rapid heartbeat or palpitations
- Dry mouth and unusual taste
- Diarrhea

Methylphenidate

- Dizziness and insomnia
- Seizures (rare)
- Stomach pain and rash
- Changes in blood count (like low platelets)
- Heart rhythm problems

Special Considerations for Children

Stimulants can impact growth, so children should have their height and weight monitored regularly. Some doctors recommend "medication holidays" during school breaks to assess whether the medication is still needed.

Nursing Process

Assessment

- Review the patient's full medical history—especially for heart conditions, high blood pressure, or hyperthyroidism.
- Monitor sleep patterns and check for adverse effects like overstimulation or mood changes.
- Talk with patients and families to ensure they understand how and when to take the medication.

Key Nursing Diagnoses

- Ineffective health maintenance due to ADHD
- Insomnia related to stimulant use
- Deficient knowledge regarding medication

Planning Goals

- Improved focus and decreased hyperactivity
- Better sleep with minimal side effects
- Patient and family understand how to use the medication safely

Implementation Tips

- Administer stimulants early in the day (at least 6 hours before bedtime) to prevent sleep issues.
- Gradually taper the dose after long-term use to avoid rebound depression.
- Educate the patient to avoid caffeine, which can amplify stimulant side effects.
- Alert the prescriber if side effects worsen or the medication loses effectiveness.

- Encourage regular check-ins to assess growth, heart rate, and blood pressure (especially in kids).

Evaluation

- Patient shows improvement in focus, behavior, or wakefulness.
- No signs of sleep disturbance or overstimulation.
- Patient and family demonstrate understanding of safe and proper use of the medication.

Chapter 12: Anti-infective Medicines

12.1. Medications for Infections

When an infection invades the body, medications known as anti-infective drugs become critical allies in fighting off harmful microorganisms. There are several key categories:

- Antibacterial drugs for bacterial infections
- Antiviral drugs for viral infections
- Antitubercular medications specifically targeting tuberculosis
- Antifungal drugs to combat fungal infections
- Other specialized medications such as antiprotozoals and antiparasitics for specific types of infections

Choosing the Right Medication

Selecting the correct anti-infective medication involves careful consideration of several factors:

- Identify the microorganism: Typically done by taking a sample and growing it in a laboratory culture.
- Determine drug sensitivity: Laboratory testing reveals which medication the microorganism is most vulnerable to. This process, known as culture and sensitivity testing, usually takes around 48 hours. However, treatment generally starts immediately, with adjustments made based on these test results.
- Infection location: The medication must effectively reach the site of infection in sufficient concentration to be successful.
- Safety and cost considerations: It's important to choose medications that are affordable, have manageable side effects, and do not trigger allergic reactions in the patient.

Preventing Drug Resistance

Over time, microorganisms can develop ways to resist medications, making infections harder to treat.

How Resistance Happens

Resistance occurs when microorganisms genetically mutate, enabling them to survive despite the presence of medication designed to eliminate them. Preventing resistance requires careful selection and appropriate use of anti-infective medications.

12.2. Antibacterial Drug

Antibacterial medications, commonly known as antibiotics, help your body fight bacterial infections by either killing bacteria or preventing their growth. They're especially important for treating systemic infections—those that affect the whole body rather than just one small area. Some main categories of antibiotics include:

- Aminoglycosides
- Penicillins
- Cephalosporins
- Tetracyclines
- Clindamycin (Cleocin)
- Macrolides
- Vancomycin (Vancocin)
- Carbapenems
- Monobactams
- Fluoroquinolones
- Sulfonamides
- Nitrofurantoin
- Linezolid (Zyvox)

Aminoglycosides

What They Do:

Aminoglycosides eliminate bacteria by directly killing them. They're particularly effective against certain types of infections caused by:

- Gram-negative bacteria
- Some gram-positive aerobic bacteria
- Mycobacteria
- Certain protozoa

Commonly Used Aminoglycosides:

- Amikacin (Amikin)
- Gentamicin (Garamycin)
- Kanamycin (Kantrex)
- Neomycin (Neo-Fradin)
- Paromomycin (Humatin)
- Streptomycin (Streptomycin)
- Tobramycin (Nebcin)

How They Move in Your Body:

Aminoglycosides don't absorb well from your digestive system, so they're typically given through an IV or as injections. The exception is neomycin, which is taken orally before certain surgeries to cleanse the bowel. These drugs spread through your body's extracellular fluid and can cross the placenta, but they don't easily enter your brain.

Because your kidneys remove these drugs, kidney health is important. Reduced kidney function can mean these drugs stay in your body longer.

How They Work:

Aminoglycosides work by interrupting the bacteria's protein-making process, essentially preventing them from surviving.

When and How They're Used:

Doctors commonly prescribe aminoglycosides for serious infections like hospital-acquired pneumonia, severe blood infections, serious urinary tract infections, or infections that resist other medications.

They're often used with other antibiotics, such as penicillin, to treat stubborn gram-positive infections. For example, penicillin can help aminoglycosides get into bacterial cells better.

- Streptomycin is especially useful for certain mycobacterial infections, including tuberculosis.
- Neomycin helps cleanse your intestine before surgery or treat certain diarrhea conditions.

Note: Aminoglycosides don't work against anaerobic bacteria (those that live without oxygen).

Possible Interactions:

- Combining aminoglycosides with specific medications like carbenicillin or certain neuromuscular blockers may alter their effectiveness or cause breathing problems.
- Using these antibiotics with drugs like cyclosporine, amphotericin B, acyclovir, or loop diuretics increases the risk of kidney damage and hearing loss.

Potential Side Effects:

Aminoglycosides carry significant side effects, including:

- Kidney damage
- Hearing loss (which may be permanent)
- Neurological issues like numbness or muscle weakness
- Digestive discomfort (when taken orally)

Because of these risks, doctors carefully monitor your kidney function and hearing during treatment.

Penicillins

Penicillins remain among the most trusted antibiotics today. They're divided into four main groups:

- Natural penicillins (like penicillin G and penicillin V)
- Penicillinase-resistant penicillins (like dicloxacillin and nafcillin)
- Aminopenicillins (second-generation) (like amoxicillin and ampicillin)
- Broad-spectrum penicillins (like piperacillin)

How Penicillins Move in Your Body:

Penicillins taken by mouth absorb mostly in your small intestine. Absorption can vary based on the specific medication, your stomach's acidity, and whether food is present. Usually, penicillins work best if taken on an empty stomach, except for a few types like amoxicillin or amoxicillin-clavulanate (Augmentin).

Penicillins travel widely, effectively reaching tissues such as your lungs, bones, kidneys, and muscles. They leave your body mainly through urine, making them helpful for treating urinary tract infections.

How They Work:

Penicillins usually kill bacteria directly by interfering with their cell walls, weakening and destroying bacterial cells.

When and How They're Used:

Penicillins are broadly effective antibiotics that target many infections, covering gram-positive, gram-negative, and anaerobic bacteria. Different types of penicillins work best against specific bacteria, and doctors choose based on your particular infection.

Nursing Care: Keeping You Safe

When you're prescribed aminoglycosides or penicillins, nurses typically:

- Carefully assess your medical history, especially allergies.

- Regularly test your kidney function and hearing, especially when taking aminoglycosides.
- Monitor you for interactions with other medications you might be taking.
- Help ensure you remain hydrated to protect your kidneys.
- Educate you and your family about how to take the medications safely and what side effects to watch for.

Penicillin: A Versatile Antibiotic

Sometimes, oral administration of penicillin isn't practical—such as when patients might struggle to consistently take pills. In these cases, intramuscular (IM) injections become a valuable alternative. Certain types, like penicillin G benzathine and penicillin G procaine, are long-acting but not easily soluble, so they must be given through IM injections.

Potential Drug Interactions

Penicillin may interact with other medications in several ways:

- Probenecid: Increases the levels of penicillin in the bloodstream.
- Methotrexate: Penicillin can reduce methotrexate clearance, increasing toxicity.
- Tetracyclines and Chloramphenicol: May decrease penicillin's effectiveness.
- Neomycin: Can reduce absorption of penicillin V.
- Hormonal Contraceptives: Penicillin V and ampicillin can lower contraceptive effectiveness. Advise patients to use additional birth control methods during therapy.
- Anticoagulants: Large IV doses of penicillin may increase bleeding risks, and certain penicillins can interfere with warfarin effectiveness.
- Electrolyte Imbalances: Penicillin may worsen hyperkalemia (high potassium) or hypernatremia (high sodium).

- Aminoglycosides and Clavulanic Acid: Can enhance the effectiveness of penicillin.

Adverse Reactions to Penicillin

Penicillin can cause several adverse reactions, notably allergic responses, which include:

- Severe allergic reactions (anaphylaxis)
- Serum sickness (fever, rash, joint pain, after injection)
- Drug fever
- Skin rashes

Digestive reactions might include:

- Oral yeast infections
- Nausea and vomiting
- Diarrhea

Neurological symptoms occasionally occur, including:

- Fatigue or lethargy
- Hallucinations
- Anxiety, depression, or confusion
- Seizures

Additionally, some types of penicillin can cause severe diarrhea known as pseudomembranous colitis, typically due to bacterial overgrowth in the colon.

Nursing Considerations with Penicillin Therapy

Assessment:

- Gather a detailed allergy history to distinguish between true allergies and mild adverse effects.
- Obtain infection cultures before therapy starts and monitor regularly to evaluate effectiveness.
- Keep an eye on vital signs, kidney function, electrolytes, and neurological status.

- Monitor blood clotting parameters, especially in high-dose or prolonged treatments.
- Evaluate patient and family understanding of the medication.

Nursing Diagnoses:

- Risk for further infection
- Risk of dehydration due to gastrointestinal reactions
- Lack of patient knowledge regarding medication

Goals of Treatment:

- Resolution of the infection, shown by normal lab results and improved symptoms.
- Maintenance of proper hydration.
- Effective education for the patient and family regarding medication use.

Implementation Tips:

- Administer penicillin at least an hour before certain antibiotics like tetracyclines or erythromycin.
- Give oral penicillin doses on an empty stomach to enhance absorption, except when specifically instructed otherwise.
- Properly store and administer oral suspensions, shaking well before use.
- Administer IM injections deep into muscle and rotate injection sites to minimize discomfort.
- Avoid mixing other medications in IV lines with penicillin, especially aminoglycosides.
- Closely monitor for allergic reactions, even if the patient has previously tolerated penicillin.
- Watch hydration status closely, particularly with gastrointestinal side effects.

Evaluation:

- Infection resolves completely.

- Adequate hydration is maintained.
- Patient and family demonstrate understanding of medication.

Cephalosporins: Broad and Effective

Cephalosporins, a widely-used group of antibiotics, are classified into generations based on effectiveness and development history:

- First-generation: Effective mostly against gram-positive bacteria; often substitutes for patients allergic to penicillin.
- Second-generation: Broader activity against gram-negative bacteria and certain anaerobes.
- Third-generation: Primarily target serious gram-negative infections.
- Fourth-generation: Active against a broad spectrum of both gram-positive and negative bacteria.
- Fifth-generation: Designed for highly resistant bacterial strains.

Interactions and Precautions:

- Alcohol consumption while taking certain cephalosporins can cause severe reactions (flushing, nausea, vomiting).
- Gout medications (probenecid, sulfinpyrazone) can affect cephalosporin levels in the body.

Side Effects and Risks:

Common adverse reactions include:

- Confusion and seizures (rare)
- Increased bleeding risk, particularly with cefotetan and ceftriaxone
- Digestive upset: nausea, vomiting, diarrhea
- Allergic reactions such as rash, itching, or, rarely, severe allergic responses

Nursing Considerations for Cephalosporins:

- Confirm allergy history before starting treatment.

- Monitor continuously for allergic and adverse reactions.
- Collect culture specimens before initiating therapy to ensure proper antibiotic selection.
- Ensure proper medication administration guidelines, storage, and IV site care.
- Regularly assess kidney function, clotting parameters, and signs of possible superinfection.

Tetracyclines: Broad-Spectrum Antibiotics

Tetracyclines are a group of antibiotics known for their wide range of antibacterial activity. They're usually classified based on how long they act in the body:

- Intermediate-acting: demeclocycline (Declomycin), tetracycline (Achromycin)
- Long-acting: doxycycline (Vibramycin), minocycline (Minocin)

How They Work in the Body (Pharmacokinetics)

When taken by mouth, tetracyclines are absorbed in the upper part of the small intestine (duodenum). They spread throughout body tissues and fluids, with high concentrations found in bile.

Most tetracyclines leave the body through the kidneys, although doxycycline is also excreted in feces. Minocycline has a recycling process through the liver and intestines (enterohepatic recirculation), which helps it stay active longer.

How They Fight Bacteria (Pharmacodynamics)

Tetracyclines don't kill bacteria outright—they stop them from growing by preventing the bacteria from making essential proteins. They get inside the bacterial cell using energy and then attach to the ribosome (the cell's protein factory) to block protein synthesis.

The long-acting types, doxycycline and minocycline, tend to be more effective against a broader range of bugs.

When They're Used (Pharmacotherapeutics)

These antibiotics can treat a wide variety of infections caused by:

- Gram-positive and gram-negative bacteria (both aerobic and anaerobic)
- Spirochetes
- Mycoplasma
- Rickettsia
- Chlamydia
- Gonorrhea
- Some protozoal infections

Common conditions treated with tetracyclines include:

- Rocky Mountain spotted fever
- Q fever
- Lyme disease
- Certain types of urethritis (especially from Chlamydia and Ureaplasma)

For brucellosis, tetracyclines are paired with streptomycin for the most effective treatment.

Low doses of tetracyclines are also effective for acne, helping reduce the fatty acids in sebum and decreasing inflammation.

Important Drug Interactions

Tetracyclines can interfere with other medications and substances:

- They can reduce the effectiveness of birth control pills, so patients should use backup contraception.
- They may also weaken the effect of penicillin.
- Antacids with aluminum, calcium, or magnesium—as well as iron, zinc, and bismuth—can block tetracycline absorption. Space them 2 to 3 hours apart.
- Drugs like barbiturates, carbamazepine, and phenytoin speed up how fast the body breaks down doxycycline, reducing its effect.

Dairy products (except with doxycycline and minocycline) can also interfere with absorption. It's best to take tetracyclines 1 hour before or 2 hours after meals.

Lifestyle Tips

- Avoid sun exposure—tetracyclines can make your skin extra sensitive to light.
- Skip alcohol while on doxycycline—it can reduce the drug's effectiveness.

Side Effects

- Like many antibiotics, tetracyclines can cause:
- Nausea, vomiting, stomach upset, diarrhea
- Superinfections (like oral thrush or yeast infections)
- Skin sensitivity to sunlight (rash, redness)
- Liver or kidney problems
- Tooth discoloration and enamel defects in children or if taken during pregnancy
- Possible effects on fetal bone development

Nursing Considerations for Tetracyclines

Assessment

- Always check for allergies first.
- Monitor for side effects, especially in elderly or immunocompromised patients.
- Get cultures before starting treatment—then monitor the response.

Nursing Diagnoses

- Risk for infection
- Risk for fluid loss (from GI side effects)
- Knowledge gap about medication

Goals

- Infection clears up (improved lab results, normal temperature)
- Fluid balance stays normal
- Patient and family understand how to take the medication

Implementation Tips

- Give oral tetracyclines (except doxycycline and minocycline) on an empty stomach.
- Don't mix them with milk, antacids, or iron supplements.
- Give with a full glass of water and keep the patient upright for 30 minutes to avoid throat irritation.
- Don't give right before bed.
- Watch expiration dates—expired tetracyclines can damage kidneys.
- Keep an eye out for superinfections or signs of local irritation with IV use.

Evaluation

- Infection resolved
- Hydration maintained
- Patient understands their treatment

Clindamycin (Cleocin): A Powerful Option—With Caution

Clindamycin is a strong antibiotic derived from lincomycin. It's often reserved for serious infections when other, safer options aren't available or when the patient is allergic to penicillin.

Pharmacokinetics

It's well absorbed when taken orally and spreads widely through the body. It's processed by the liver and leaves the body through both urine and bile.

How It Works

Like tetracyclines, clindamycin blocks protein synthesis in bacteria. It's mainly bacteriostatic, meaning it slows down bacterial growth rather than killing bacteria outright.

When It's Used

Because of the risk of serious side effects—especially pseudomembranous colitis (a dangerous type of severe diarrhea)—clindamycin is only used in select cases:

- Works against most gram-positive bacteria and anaerobes
- Treats abdominal, lung, and other infections caused by Bacteroides fragilis
- Can treat Clostridium perfringens infections when penicillin can't be used
- An alternative for staph infections in penicillin-allergic patients

Drug Interactions

- May increase the effects of neuromuscular blockers, risking respiratory problems
- Don't combine with erythromycin—they compete for the same binding sites

Side Effects

- Most serious: Pseudomembranous colitis, which can be fatal if untreated
- Others: Diarrhea, mouth irritation, nausea, vomiting, allergic reactions

Nursing Considerations for Clindamycin

Assessment

- Monitor liver, kidney, and blood function during long-term use
- Watch for early signs of GI side effects
- Get culture and sensitivity tests before starting therapy

Planning and Goals

- Infection resolves
- Fluids stay balanced
- Patient and family understand the medication and its risks

Implementation

- Don't refrigerate the oral solution—it thickens and becomes hard to use
- Give capsules with a full glass of water
- IM injections can be painful—rotate sites and limit to 600 mg per injection
- Monitor IV sites for phlebitis
- Never use opioids for clindamycin-induced diarrhea—it can make things worse

Evaluation

- Infection under control
- No severe side effects
- Patient understands proper use and precautions

Macrolides: Versatile Antibiotics

Macrolides are commonly used to treat respiratory infections and others. This class includes:

- Erythromycin (Pediamycin, Erythrocin, Bristamycin)
- Azithromycin (Zmax)
- Clarithromycin (Biaxin)
- Fidaxomicin (Dificid)
- Telithromycin (Ketek)

Pharmacokinetics

- Erythromycin is sensitive to stomach acid, so it's often coated or buffered. It's absorbed in the duodenum and distributed widely, except to the CSF—unless the meninges are inflamed.

- Erythromycin is mostly eliminated via bile.
- Azithromycin and clarithromycin are absorbed quickly and spread through most tissues, but don't enter the CNS well. Azithromycin is also excreted in bile; clarithromycin goes mostly through urine.
- Fidaxomicin stays in the GI tract and is excreted in feces, while telithromycin is metabolized by the liver.

How They Work

- Macrolides stop bacterial protein synthesis by acting on the ribosome, similar to clindamycin.

Uses

- Effective against many gram-positive and gram-negative organisms
- Treat infections caused by Mycoplasma, Treponema, Chlamydia, and Streptococcus
- First-line for Mycoplasma pneumoniae and Legionella
- Fidaxomicin is specifically for C. difficile infections
- Telithromycin is used for community-acquired pneumonia, including drug-resistant strains

In penicillin-allergic patients, macrolides like erythromycin offer a solid alternative for strep, pneumonia, gonorrhea, syphilis, and minor staph infections.

Macrolides: Applause for the Broad-Spectrum Stars

Macrolides are known for their wide-ranging ability to tackle many different bacterial infections—making them true "broad-spectrum" antibiotics.

Who's Who in the Macrolide Lineup

- Azithromycin steps up with strong activity against both gram-positive and gram-negative bacteria—including Mycobacterium,

306

Staphylococcus aureus, Haemophilus influenzae, Moraxella catarrhalis, and Chlamydia. It's also effective against pneumococci and group C, F, and G streptococci.

- Clarithromycin is another broad-acting option. It works against gram-positive bacteria like S. aureus, S. pneumoniae, and S. pyogenes, as well as gram-negative types like H. influenzae and M. catarrhalis. It also hits other bugs like Mycoplasma pneumoniae.
- Clarithromycin also shines when used alongside other medications—like antacids, H2 blockers, and proton pump inhibitors—to treat Helicobacter pylori–related duodenal ulcers.

Drug Interactions: Proceed with Caution

While macrolides are generally well-tolerated, they can interact with other medications:

- Erythromycin, azithromycin, and clarithromycin may raise the levels of theophylline, increasing the risk of toxicity—especially at higher doses.
- Clarithromycin can also boost carbamazepine levels.
- Telithromycin is metabolized through the CYP3A4 liver pathway and may cause serious interactions—especially with colchicine in patients with kidney or liver issues.
- Avoid using telithromycin with cisapride or pimozide, as this combo may dangerously extend the QT interval on an ECG.
- Fidaxomicin shouldn't be combined with cyclosporine due to potential complications.

Common Adverse Reactions

Macrolides typically have a low side-effect profile, but they can still cause:

- Upset stomach (epigastric distress), nausea, vomiting
- Diarrhea (especially at higher doses)
- Skin rashes, fever

- Increased eosinophils (a type of white blood cell)
- Rarely, anaphylaxis

Nursing Process: Caring for Patients on Macrolides

Assessment

- Evaluate the infection before and during treatment.
- Always obtain culture and sensitivity results before starting.
- Watch for any signs of adverse reactions or drug interactions.
- Assess the patient's and family's understanding of the medication.

Nursing Diagnoses

- Risk for infection due to altered immune response
- Risk for fluid loss from GI side effects
- Knowledge gap regarding drug use and safety

Planning Goals

- Infection improves (as seen in lab tests and vitals)
- Fluid balance stays within normal limits
- Patient and family understand how and why the medication is being used

Implementation Tips

- For suspensions, double-check the concentration.
- Give oral macrolides 1 hour before or 2 hours after meals with a full glass of water (unless coated tablets are used—those can be taken with food).
- Avoid giving the drug with fruit juice.
- Chewable erythromycin tablets should be chewed—not swallowed whole.
- Coated tablets or encapsulated forms often cause less stomach upset.

- Follow reconstitution instructions precisely. For IV doses, dilute 250 mg in at least 100 mL of normal saline and infuse over 1 hour.
- Avoid mixing erythromycin lactobionate with other IV drugs.
- Monitor liver function—macrolides can raise liver enzymes and may cause liver damage in rare cases.
- If GI issues arise, monitor hydration and electrolyte balance.

Evaluation

- Infection resolves
- Hydration maintained
- Patient and family demonstrate good understanding of medication use

Vancomycin: A Heavy Hitter Against Tough Bugs

Vancomycin is a go-to drug when facing serious infections—especially methicillin-resistant Staphylococcus aureus (MRSA). Because of growing concerns about vancomycin-resistant enterococci (VRE), its use should be reserved for cases where it's truly needed and confirmed by culture results.

How It Moves in the Body (Pharmacokinetics)

Vancomycin is poorly absorbed from the GI tract, so it's usually given by IV for serious systemic infections. The oral form is reserved for C. difficile colitis—not interchangeable with the IV form.

Once in the bloodstream, vancomycin spreads well to many areas, including the lungs, heart sac, joints, and abdominal cavity.

Most of it—around 85%—is excreted unchanged in the urine within 24 hours. A small amount may leave the body through the liver and bile.

How It Works (Pharmacodynamics)

Vancomycin attacks bacteria by stopping them from building their cell walls, which weakens them and allows the immune system to take over.

What It Treats (Pharmacotherapeutics)

Targets gram-positive aerobic organisms like S. aureus, S. epidermidis, S. pyogenes, Enterococcus, and S. pneumoniae.

- IV form is used for serious staph infections when patients are allergic to penicillin.
- Oral form is effective against antibiotic-associated colitis, especially from C. difficile.
- When combined with an aminoglycoside, it treats E. faecalis endocarditis in penicillin-allergic patients.

Drug Interactions to Know

Vancomycin can be toxic to the kidneys and ears, especially when given with:

- Aminoglycosides
- Amphotericin B
- Cisplatin
- Bacitracin
- Colistin
- Polymyxin B

Adverse Reactions

While rare, serious reactions include:

- Hypersensitivity or anaphylaxis
- Drug fever
- Increased eosinophils or decreased neutrophils
- Hearing loss (especially with high doses or when paired with other ototoxic drugs)
- Kidney damage
- Red man syndrome: a rash, flushing, and low blood pressure if the drug is infused too quickly

Pro tip: Infuse 1 g of vancomycin over at least 1 hour. For doses above 1 g, take 1.5–2 hours to prevent red man syndrome.

Nursing Process for Vancomycin

Assessment

- Evaluate infection regularly and get cultures before starting.
- Get baseline hearing and kidney function tests—and monitor during treatment.
- Monitor serum drug levels, especially in neonates, elderly patients, or those with kidney disease.
- Watch for interactions and adverse reactions.

Diagnoses

- Risk for infection
- Risk for dehydration from GI issues
- Knowledge deficit about treatment

Goals

- Infection clears up
- Fluid balance maintained
- Patient/family understand the therapy and precautions

Implementation Tips

- Adjust dose for patients with kidney problems.
- Don't give the drug by IM injection.
- Oral form stays stable in the fridge for 2 weeks.
- Infuse IV form in 200 mL of D5W over 60 minutes.
- Check IV sites daily for irritation or signs of tissue damage.
- If red man syndrome occurs, stop the infusion immediately and notify the provider.
- Store IV solutions in the fridge and use within 96 hours.
- For staph endocarditis, treatment usually lasts at least 4 weeks.

Evaluation

- Infection resolved
- Hydration maintained

- Understanding of medication confirmed

Carbapenems: The Big Guns of Antibiotics

Carbapenems are powerful beta-lactam antibiotics used to treat serious, hospital-acquired infections. This class includes:

- Imipenem-cilastatin (Primaxin)
- Meropenem (Merrem)
- Ertapenem (Invanz)
- Doripenem (Doribax)

How They Work in the Body

- Imipenem must be paired with cilastatin, which prevents it from being broken down by the kidneys too quickly.
- Ertapenem is highly protein-bound and excreted mostly in the urine.
- Meropenem spreads widely—including to the brain—and is mostly excreted unchanged in the urine.

Mechanism of Action

Carbapenems kill bacteria by preventing them from building their cell walls.

What They Treat

- Imipenem-cilastatin has the widest range—effective against gram-positive and gram-negative bacteria, including Pseudomonas and Bacteroides fragilis.
- Meropenem treats intra-abdominal infections and bacterial meningitis.
- Ertapenem covers infections in the abdomen, urinary tract, skin, and lungs.
- Doripenem is approved for complicated UTIs and intra-abdominal infections in adults.

Drug Interactions

- Probenecid can increase the blood levels of carbapenems—raising the risk of side effects.
- Imipenem-cilastatin + aminoglycosides = synergistic action against E. faecalis.

Adverse Reactions

Common ones include:

- Nausea, vomiting, diarrhea
- Allergic reactions (especially in patients allergic to penicillin)

Ertapenem may also cause:

- Seizures
- Low blood pressure
- High potassium
- Trouble breathing
- Rarely, death

Nursing Process for Carbapenems

Assessment

- Monitor infection status regularly
- Get cultures before starting
- Watch for side effects or interactions
- Assess the patient's knowledge and hydration

Diagnoses

- Risk for infection
- Risk for fluid imbalance
- Lack of knowledge about therapy

Goals

- Clear infection
- Maintain fluid balance

- Patient/family understand the treatment plan

Implementation Tips

- Never give by direct IV bolus—always infuse over 40–60 minutes
- If nausea occurs, slow the infusion rate
- Use lidocaine (without epinephrine) for IM injections
- Solutions are stable for 10 hours at room temp or 48 hours refrigerated
- Adjust dosing in kidney impairment
- If seizures occur, notify the prescriber and initiate seizure precautions

Evaluation

- Infection under control
- No dehydration or fluid imbalance
- Patient and family understand medication use

Monobactams: When Penicillin's Off the Table

Monobactams are a unique class of antibiotics, designed especially for patients who are allergic to penicillins. They work similarly to other antibiotics—by binding to bacterial enzymes and disrupting cell wall synthesis—but their structure sets them apart.

Meet the MVP: Aztreonam (Azactam)

Aztreonam is the only monobactam currently in use. It's synthetic, and it has a narrow—but focused—spectrum, mainly targeting gram-negative aerobic bacteria.

How It Moves Through the Body (Pharmacokinetics)

When given via injection or IV, aztreonam is quickly and completely absorbed, spreading well throughout the body. It's only partially broken down and is mostly excreted through the urine in its original form.

How It Works (Pharmacodynamics)

Aztreonam is bactericidal—it kills bacteria by stopping them from building strong cell walls. It targets a specific protein (PBP-3) on gram-negative bacteria, which leads to cell wall breakdown and bacterial death.

When It's Used (Pharmacotherapeutics)

Aztreonam is effective in treating:

- UTIs (complicated and uncomplicated)
- Septicemia
- Lower respiratory tract infections
- Skin and soft tissue infections
- Intra-abdominal and gynecologic infections

It's often used when bacteria produce beta-lactamase, an enzyme that destroys other antibiotics. Aztreonam is resistant to that trick.

Important: Aztreonam should not be used alone in seriously ill patients if there's a chance of gram-positive or mixed infections. It's not a catch-all—use it wisely.

Drug Interactions to Watch

- Probenecid can increase aztreonam levels by slowing its excretion.
- Synergistic effects can occur with drugs like aminoglycosides, cefoperazone, cefotaxime, clindamycin, and piperacillin.
- Avoid combining with cefoxitin or imipenem—these can actually inactivate aztreonam.
- Results may vary with clavulanic acid–containing antibiotics—effects could be helpful or harmful, depending on the bug.

Adverse Reactions

Watch out for:

- Diarrhea, nausea, vomiting

- Low blood pressure
- Skin reactions or allergic responses
- Temporary changes on ECG (like arrhythmias)
- Slight increases in liver enzymes

Nursing Considerations

Assessment

- Monitor infection signs regularly
- Get cultures before starting treatment
- Watch for drug reactions or allergic responses
- Gauge patient/family understanding

Diagnoses

- Risk for infection
- Risk for fluid loss from GI side effects
- Knowledge gap about drug therapy

Planning Goals

- Infection clears up
- Fluid levels remain stable
- Patient and family understand treatment plan

Implementation

- Even if a patient is allergic to penicillin, aztreonam is usually safe—but still, watch closely.
- For IV bolus, inject slowly over 3–5 minutes.
- Infusions should run over 20–60 minutes.
- For IM injections, go deep—use a large muscle like the gluteus or thigh. Let the patient know there may be swelling or discomfort.
- Doses over 1 gram should be given IV, not IM.

Evaluation

- Infection resolved

- Hydration intact
- Patient and family show understanding

Fluoroquinolones: Fast, Broad, and Powerful

Fluoroquinolones are synthetic antibiotics used for a wide range of infections—especially urinary tract infections (UTIs), respiratory infections, pneumonia, and gonorrhea.

Common Drugs in This Class

- Ciprofloxacin (Cipro)
- Levofloxacin (Levaquin)
- Moxifloxacin (Avelox)
- Norfloxacin (Noroxin)
- Ofloxacin (Floxin)
- Gemifloxacin (Factive)

Pharmacokinetics

- Absorption: Excellent when taken orally
- Metabolism: Minimal liver metabolism
- Excretion: Mainly through urine
- Protein binding: Low

Pharmacodynamics: How They Work

These drugs block DNA gyrase, an enzyme bacteria need to replicate. Without it, bacteria can't reproduce—making fluoroquinolones bactericidal.

What They Treat

Each drug has its own specialty:

- Ciprofloxacin: Lower respiratory infections, infectious diarrhea, bone/skin/joint infections
- Levofloxacin: UTIs, skin infections, lower respiratory infections
- Moxifloxacin: Sinus infections, community-acquired pneumonia

- Norfloxacin: UTIs and prostatitis
- Ofloxacin: STIs, respiratory and skin infections, prostatitis; also available in ear and eye drop forms
- Gemifloxacin: Bronchitis flares and mild pneumonia

Drug Interactions

- Antacids (with aluminum or magnesium) interfere with absorption
- Theophylline and fluoroquinolones can interact, increasing the risk of toxicity
- Probenecid slows elimination, increasing drug levels
- Be cautious with QT-prolonging drugs (like antiarrhythmics) while taking moxifloxacin

Adverse Effects

Most people tolerate fluoroquinolones well, but side effects can include:

- Dizziness, nausea, vomiting
- Diarrhea, abdominal pain
- Tendinitis and tendon rupture
- Blurred vision, tinnitus
- Fever, chills

Caution with sunlight! Fluoroquinolones can cause phototoxicity, even with sunscreen. Patients should avoid sun and UV exposure during and shortly after treatment.

Nursing Considerations

Assessment

- Monitor infection status
- Get cultures before starting therapy
- Watch for reactions or side effects
- Assess understanding of treatment

Diagnoses

- Infection risk
- Fluid imbalance from GI effects
- Deficient knowledge about the drug

Goals

- Infection resolves
- Fluid levels stay normal
- Patient and family understand medication

Implementation

- Oral doses: 2 hours before/after meals, and at least 6 hours apart from antacids, sucralfate, or iron
- Dilute IV doses as directed; infuse over 1 hour into a large vein
- Adjust dosage for kidney problems
- Watch hydration if GI symptoms arise

Evaluation

- Infection resolved
- No signs of dehydration
- Patient/family demonstrate understanding

Sulfonamides: Old but Still Gold

Sulfonamides were among the first systemic antibiotics ever used—and they're still relevant today.

Common Sulfonamides

- Trimethoprim + Sulfamethoxazole (Bactrim)
- Sulfadiazine (Silvadene)
- Sulfasalazine (Azulfidine)

Pharmacokinetics

Well absorbed and widely distributed

Metabolized in the liver, excreted through the kidneys

Important: Drink plenty of fluids to avoid crystal formation in urine

How They Work (Pharmacodynamics)

Sulfonamides are bacteriostatic—they stop bacteria from growing by blocking folic acid synthesis, which bacteria need to make DNA and multiply.

What They Treat

- Most commonly used for acute UTIs
- Also effective against Nocardia asteroides and Toxoplasma gondii
- Effective against a broad range of gram-positive and gram-negative bacteria

Combination Therapy

The combo drug trimethoprim-sulfamethoxazole is often used for:

- Pneumocystis carinii pneumonia
- Ear infections (acute otitis media)
- Chronic bronchitis flares

Drug Interactions

- Increases the effects of sulfonylureas (can cause low blood sugar)
- Can lead to urine crystals if taken with methenamine
- May increase the action of coumarin anticoagulants
- Risk of kidney damage when combined with cyclosporine

Adverse Effects

- Crystalluria (crystals in urine)—especially with older drugs or poor hydration
- Hypersensitivity reactions (rash, fever, joint pain)
- Photosensitivity
- Serum sickness–like symptoms (hives, joint pain, leukopenia)

Nursing Considerations

Assessment

- Review allergy history, especially to sulfa drugs
- Check for signs of infection and side effects
- Monitor kidney function, CBC, and urine output
- Get cultures before starting

Diagnoses

- Risk for infection
- Risk of dehydration or superinfection
- Deficient knowledge of medication

Goals

- Infection resolves
- Fluid and electrolyte balance maintained
- Patient/family understand treatment

Implementation

- Give oral doses with at least 8 oz of water
- Encourage 3–4 liters of fluid per day
- Ensure minimum urine output of 1,500 mL/day
- Shake suspensions well before use
- Follow instructions for reconstituting and storing

Evaluation

- Patient is infection-free
- Hydration is stable
- Patient and family can explain medication use

Nitrofurantoin (Furadantin): Targeting UTIs at the Source

Nitrofurantoin is a well-known antibiotic used to treat both acute and chronic urinary tract infections (UTIs). What makes it especially effective? It works best in acidic urine, which is common in many UTI cases.

How It's Absorbed and Processed (Pharmacokinetics)

Nitrofurantoin is rapidly absorbed from the GI tract after oral administration—and taking it with food makes it work even better.

Form Matters

There are two forms:

- Microcrystalline: Absorbed more slowly, so it tends to cause less stomach upset.
- Macrocrystalline: Often easier on the gut.

Where It Goes in the Body

- 20–60% protein-bound
- Crosses the placenta and appears in breast milk
- Also found in bile
- Partially broken down by the liver
- Around 30–50% is excreted unchanged in urine

How It Works (Pharmacodynamics)

Nitrofurantoin is bacteriostatic at lower concentrations—meaning it stops bacteria from multiplying. At higher concentrations, especially in the urine, it can become bactericidal, directly killing the bacteria.

Even though the exact mechanism isn't fully understood, it appears to block bacterial energy production and may also mess with the cell wall.

When It's Used (Pharmacotherapeutics)

Nitrofurantoin is effective only in the urinary tract, not for systemic infections. It's a great option for:

- Uncomplicated UTIs
- Long-term suppression of chronic UTIs

Not for kidney-related infections! It won't help with pyelonephritis or infections around the kidneys (perinephric infections).

Drug Interactions

Nitrofurantoin doesn't have many major interactions, but keep these in mind:

- Probenecid and sulfinpyrazone can block excretion, making the drug less effective and more toxic.
- Magnesium-based antacids can reduce absorption.
- May reduce the effectiveness of norfloxacin and nalidixic acid.

Adverse Reactions

Some people experience:

- GI upset: nausea, vomiting, anorexia, abdominal pain
- Dark yellow or brown urine (harmless, but alarming to some patients)
- Chills, fever, joint pain
- Allergic reactions, including skin, blood, liver, or lung involvement
- Rare but serious: anaphylaxis

Nursing Process: Nitrofurantoin

Assessment

- Check infection signs before and during therapy.
- Review allergy history, especially to sulfa drugs or other sulfur-containing meds.
- Monitor for drug reactions and side effects.
- Get cultures before the first dose and check effectiveness over time.
- Talk with the patient and family to assess their understanding.

Key Nursing Diagnoses

- Risk for infection due to resistance or superinfection

- Risk for fluid loss due to GI symptoms
- Lack of knowledge about how and when to take the drug

Planning Goals

- Infection improves (labs and symptoms normalize)
- Patient stays well hydrated
- Patient/family can explain how to take the medication properly

Implementation

- Give with food or milk to ease stomach issues
- Monitor for hypersensitivity
- Continue therapy 3 days after urine is sterile
- Watch for changes in pulmonary function or CBC
- Monitor fluid intake/output
- Reassure patients that urine color changes are expected

Evaluation

- Patient is free from infection
- Hydration is maintained
- Patient and family understand and adhere to treatment

Linezolid (Zyvox): A Precision Antibiotic for Resistant Infections

Linezolid is a synthetic antibiotic from the oxazolidinone class. It's a strong, targeted treatment, particularly effective against resistant gram-positive infections, and sometimes used against select gram-negative or anaerobic bugs.

How It Moves Through the Body (Pharmacokinetics)

Linezolid can be taken orally or via IV, and it absorbs well regardless of food. It spreads easily into body tissues.

- Its metabolism is minimal and not fully mapped out.

- Excretion mostly occurs via non-renal routes (outside the kidneys).

ow It Works (Pharmacodynamics)

Linezolid blocks bacterial protein synthesis by attaching to bacterial RNA. This prevents bacteria from building the materials they need to reproduce.

When It's Used (Pharmacotherapeutics)

Linezolid is a powerful option against:

- Vancomycin-resistant Enterococcus faecium (VRE)
- Methicillin-resistant Staph aureus (MRSA)
- Streptococcus species (including pneumoniae, pyogenes, agalactiae)

Used for:

- Hospital-acquired (nosocomial) pneumonia

- Community-acquired pneumonia
- Complicated and uncomplicated skin infections
- Does not treat osteomyelitis unless specifically indicated.

Drug Interactions

Linezolid is a reversible, non-selective MAO inhibitor. That means:

- Don't give with MAO inhibitors or within 2 weeks of taking one.
- Use with extreme caution in patients on serotonin-based antidepressants. There's a risk of serotonin syndrome, a potentially life-threatening condition. If no alternative exists, stop the antidepressant and monitor closely.

Adverse Effects

Most common side effects include:

- Headache, diarrhea, nausea, vomiting
- Anemia, thrombocytopenia, leukopenia, or pancytopenia (especially with long-term use)
- Peripheral or optic neuropathy with treatment lasting longer than 28 days
- Hypersensitivity reactions

Nursing Process: Linezolid

Assessment

- Evaluate the infection before and during treatment
- Get culture and sensitivity results before starting
- Watch for adverse reactions (especially blood-related) and serotonin syndrome risks
- Assess hydration and patient knowledge

Key Diagnoses

- Risk for infection due to resistance
- Risk for dehydration from GI symptoms
- Deficient knowledge about drug risks and use

Goals

- Infection is treated effectively
- Fluid status remains stable
- Patient and family understand how and when to take the drug

Implementation

- Don't refrigerate the oral suspension—it thickens. Store at room temp (good for 3 weeks)
- Inspect IV solutions before use—slight yellow tint is okay
- Check IV sites daily for phlebitis
- Infuse over 30–120 minutes
- Flush IV tubing before and after administration

- Linezolid is compatible with normal saline, D5W, and lactated Ringer's

Evaluation

- Infection resolved
- Hydration maintained
- Patient and family understand therapy and precautions

12.3. Antiviral Drugs: Defending Against Viruses Big and Small

Antiviral medications help us fight off viruses that cause everything from the common flu to complex infections like HIV and hepatitis. These drugs can either prevent viruses from multiplying or stop them from spreading within the body.

Major Classes of Systemic Antivirals

Antiviral medications fall into several groups based on how they work:

- Nucleoside analogues
- Pyrophosphate analogues
- Drugs for influenza A and respiratory syncytial virus (RSV)
- Nucleoside/nucleotide reverse transcriptase inhibitors (NRTIs)
- Non-nucleoside reverse transcriptase inhibitors (NNRTIs)
- Protease inhibitors
- Drugs for hepatitis B (HBV) and hepatitis C (HCV)

Nucleoside Analogues: Disrupting the Viral Blueprint

These drugs are commonly used in immunocompromised patients to manage viral infections like herpes simplex virus (HSV) and cytomegalovirus (CMV). Some of the most widely used drugs in this class include:

- Acyclovir (Zovirax)
- Cidofovir (Vistide)
- Famciclovir (Famvir)

- Ganciclovir (Cytovene)
- Valacyclovir (Valtrex)
- Valganciclovir (Valcyte)
- Ribavirin (Copegus) – primarily used for chronic hepatitis C and RSV (discussed under influenza/RSV)

Pharmacokinetics: How They Move Through the Body

Each drug has a unique pathway:

- Acyclovir: Orally absorbed slowly (only 15–30%). It distributes throughout the body, is mostly processed within infected cells, and exits through the urine.
- Cidofovir: Only given IV and always with probenecid, which helps reduce toxicity. Most of it is excreted unchanged by the kidneys.
- Famciclovir: Low plasma protein binding. Metabolized by the liver, excreted in urine.
- Ganciclovir: Given IV due to poor oral absorption. Over 90% is excreted unchanged by the kidneys.
- Valacyclovir: Rapidly converts to acyclovir in the body and behaves similarly.
- Valganciclovir: Metabolized to ganciclovir in the intestines and liver—not interchangeable with ganciclovir directly.

Pharmacodynamics: How They Work

These drugs generally block viral DNA synthesis:

- Acyclovir becomes acyclovir triphosphate, which blocks viral DNA polymerase—stopping virus replication.
- Cidofovir turns into cidofovir diphosphate inside cells, interfering with viral DNA without much effect on human DNA.
- Ganciclovir converts to its triphosphate form in infected cells to block viral DNA replication.

- Famciclovir inhibits DNA polymerase in HSV and varicella-zoster virus (VZV).
- Valacyclovir turns into acyclovir and works the same way.
- Valganciclovir becomes ganciclovir, primarily used for CMV.

Therapeutic Uses (Pharmacotherapeutics)

Acyclovir

Oral: Treats initial and recurrent genital herpes (HSV-2)

IV: Used for severe or widespread infections in immunocompromised patients:

- HSV type 1 or 2 (skin/mucous membrane)
- Shingles (herpes zoster)
- Disseminated chickenpox (varicella)

Other Agents

- Ganciclovir: CMV retinitis and other CMV infections in immunocompromised patients, including HIV/AIDS
- Famciclovir: Genital herpes, shingles, and herpes simplex in HIV patients
- Valacyclovir: Genital herpes, shingles, cold sores
- Cidofovir & Valganciclovir: Used for CMV retinitis in HIV patients

Key Drug Interactions

- Probenecid can raise blood levels of several antivirals (acyclovir, famciclovir, ganciclovir, valganciclovir, cidofovir), increasing risk of side effects.
- Ganciclovir + cytotoxic drugs (e.g., vincristine, amphotericin B, dapsone) can damage rapidly dividing cells (e.g., bone marrow, GI tract, skin).
- Cidofovir should not be taken with kidney-toxic drugs like aminoglycosides, NSAIDs, or amphotericin B.
- Ganciclovir + imipenem-cilastatin: Risk of seizures.

- Zidovudine + ganciclovir: Increases risk of low white blood cells—adjust dosing as needed.

Adverse Effects

- Acyclovir: Headache, nausea, diarrhea; kidney problems can occur if IV given too fast.
- Cidofovir: Kidney toxicity is common—monitor closely.
- Ganciclovir: Can cause low platelet and white cell counts (granulocytopenia, thrombocytopenia).
- Valacyclovir & famciclovir: Headache, nausea.
- Valganciclovir: May cause seizures, retinal detachment, bone marrow suppression, and neutropenia.

Nursing Process: Nucleoside Analogues

Assessment

- Evaluate the type and severity of viral infection before and during treatment.
- Watch closely for side effects and drug interactions.
- Review patient/family understanding of treatment plan.

Nursing Diagnoses

- Ineffective protection (due to bone marrow suppression)
- Risk for fluid imbalance (from GI symptoms)
- Knowledge deficit regarding drug therapy

Planning Goals

- Avoid injury and complications
- Maintain hydration
- Promote patient/family understanding

Implementation

- Monitor kidney/liver function, CBC, and platelet count
- Be alert for mental status changes (especially in patients with neurological history)

- Ensure hydration if nausea or vomiting occurs
- Administer as directed (especially for IV drugs)
- Request antiemetics/antidiarrheals if needed
- Take safety precautions for CNS side effects—bed in low position, assist with ambulation

Evaluation

- No injury or drug-related complications
- Adequate hydration maintained
- Patient and family understand therapy

Pyrophosphate Analogues: An Option for Resistant Viruses

Foscarnet (Foscavir) is a pyrophosphate analogue used when first-line antivirals aren't enough. It's especially helpful for CMV retinitis in AIDS patients and acyclovir-resistant HSV in immunocompromised patients.

Pharmacokinetics

- Poorly binds to plasma proteins
- Excreted mostly unchanged in urine in patients with normal kidney function

Pharmacodynamics

Foscarnet works by blocking DNA polymerase, preventing the virus from replicating.

Uses (Pharmacotherapeutics)

- Primary: CMV retinitis in AIDS patients
- Also used for HSV infections that don't respond to acyclovir
- Can be combined with ganciclovir for relapsed CMV

Drug Interactions

- Foscarnet + pentamidine: Raises risk of hypocalcemia and kidney damage
- Caution with other drugs that affect electrolytes
- Higher risk of nephrotoxicity with drugs like aminoglycosides or amphotericin B
- Hydration is critical to reduce kidney damage

Adverse Effects

Foscarnet has a long list of potential side effects:

- Fatigue, depression, confusion, seizures
- GI upset (nausea, vomiting, diarrhea, abdominal pain)
- Kidney damage, low calcium, phosphate, potassium
- Blood disorders: leukopenia, granulocytopenia
- Numbness, tingling, involuntary muscle contractions
- Breathing issues, skin rashes

Nursing Process: Pyrophosphate Analogues

Assessment

- Assess the infection and monitor for side effects
- Watch for drug interactions
- Review patient/family understanding

Diagnoses

- Risk for injury from hematologic or neurologic effects
- Risk for dehydration
- Deficient knowledge

Goals

- Avoid injury or CNS complications
- Maintain stable hydration
- Ensure patient/family understand treatment

Implementation

- Infuse slowly (≥1 hour) with a pump
- Hydrate well before and during infusion to protect the kidneys
- Monitor:
  Electrolytes (Ca, K, Mg, PO4)
  Creatinine clearance (2–3x weekly during initiation)
  CBC/platelets
  Mental status—watch for CNS changes
- Take safety precautions if seizures or confusion arise
- Be ready to give anti-nausea or anti-diarrheal meds
- Follow exact reconstitution/dosing instructions

Evaluation

- No serious injury or adverse effects
- Kidney function remains stable
- Patient/family show understanding of the treatment

Drugs for Influenza A & RSV: Stopping Viruses in Their Tracks

To help manage infections like influenza A and respiratory syncytial virus (RSV), we have several antiviral options. These drugs don't cure the infection, but they can shorten its course, ease symptoms, and reduce complications, especially in high-risk or immunocompromised patients.

Common Drugs in This Group:

- Oseltamivir (Tamiflu)
- Inhaled Zanamivir (Relenza)
- Peramivir (Rapivab)
- Ribavirin (Copegus, Virazole)
- Amantadine
- Rimantadine (Flumadine) — an amantadine derivative

Pharmacokinetics: How These Drugs Move Through the Body

- Amantadine, rimantadine, and oseltamivir are absorbed well when taken by mouth and widely distributed.
  Amantadine leaves the body mostly through urine.
  Rimantadine is metabolized first, then excreted in urine.
  Oseltamivir is excreted almost entirely unchanged via the kidneys.
- Ribavirin (aerosolized) and zanamivir are inhaled.
  Ribavirin builds up in the lungs and red blood cells, with variable absorption.
  Zanamivir has minimal systemic absorption and is mostly excreted unchanged in urine.
- Ribavirin (oral capsules) is well absorbed and distributed in the plasma. It's processed in the liver and RBCs, then excreted by the kidneys and feces.
- Peramivir is given IV, not metabolized much, and is mostly excreted unchanged in urine.
- Palivizumab is given as an intramuscular injection (IM). Its pharmacokinetics vary by person and are still being studied.

How They Work (Pharmacodynamics)

Each drug works a bit differently:

- Amantadine likely blocks an early stage in virus replication (exact mechanism unknown).
- Rimantadine blocks viral RNA and protein synthesis.
- Ribavirin disrupts viral RNA and DNA synthesis.
- Peramivir, oseltamivir, and zanamivir block an enzyme that helps viruses escape infected cells and spread.
- Palivizumab binds to virus proteins and blocks fusion with host cells—stopping infection before it begins.

When They're Used (Pharmacotherapeutics)

Influenza A

- Amantadine and rimantadine can both treat and prevent flu caused by influenza A.
- They help reduce symptoms, especially fever, and shorten illness duration.
- Also used to protect people who:
  Just got the flu shot (but immunity hasn't kicked in yet)
  Can't receive the vaccine due to allergies

Bonus use: Amantadine can also treat Parkinson's disease and drug-induced movement disorders.

Influenza A & B

- Oseltamivir and zanamivir treat and prevent both flu types.
- Peramivir is used only for acute treatment (not prevention) in adults.

Respiratory Syncytial Virus (RSV)

- Ribavirin is used in children with RSV and in adults with chronic hepatitis C (in combo with interferon alfa-2B).
- Palivizumab offers passive immunity to high-risk children (e.g., premature infants).

Drug Interactions

Amantadine:

- Taking it with anticholinergics can worsen side effects like dry mouth, blurred vision, or confusion.
- Diuretics (like HCTZ with triamterene) reduce amantadine excretion, raising drug levels.
- Trimethoprim increases amantadine levels too.

Rimantadine & Palivizumab

- No significant interactions known.

Ribavirin:

- Lowers the effectiveness of zidovudine (AZT)—may cause blood toxicity.
- May increase digoxin levels, risking digoxin toxicity.

Live flu vaccines (LAIV)

- Avoid using live flu vaccines 2 weeks before or 48 hours after giving oseltamivir, zanamivir, or peramivir—they can interfere with vaccine effectiveness.

Adverse Effects

Amantadine & Rimantadine (similar side effects, but rimantadine is usually milder):

- Anxiety, confusion, hallucinations, depression
- Nausea, anorexia, insomnia, irritability
- Rarely: psychosis or severe mood changes

Oseltamivir & Zanamivir:

- Headache
- Nausea, vomiting, diarrhea
- Bronchitis
- Dizziness

Peramivir & Palivizumab:

- Anaphylaxis and hypersensitivity
- Stevens-Johnson syndrome reported with peramivir

Ribavirin:

Severe reactions like:

- Apnea, cardiac arrest
- Hypotension
- Pneumothorax (collapsed lung)
- Worsened respiratory status

Nursing Process: Influenza & RSV Drugs

Assessment

- Get baseline viral infection data
- Check for side effects and any interactions
- Gauge the patient's and family's understanding of their treatment

Nursing Diagnoses

- Risk for injury (CNS or hematologic side effects)
- Risk for fluid loss (GI side effects)
- Knowledge deficit about antiviral therapy

Planning Goals

- Prevent injury or adverse reactions
- Keep hydration within normal range
- Ensure patient and family understand treatment

Implementation

- Monitor kidney/liver function, CBC, platelets
- Watch hydration—especially with vomiting or diarrhea
- In patients with heart failure, closely monitor if on amantadine
- Use safety precautions for CNS side effects: low bed, assist walking, raise rails
- Never stop amantadine abruptly in Parkinson's—it could trigger a crisis
- Reconstitute/administer per manufacturer's guidance
- Request antiemetics or antidiarrheals as needed

Evaluation

- No adverse effects or injuries during treatment
- Hydration remains stable
- Patient/family understand how to take the medication and what to watch for

NNRTIs (Non-Nucleoside Reverse Transcriptase Inhibitors)

These medications are key players in HIV therapy. They don't work alone—they're always used alongside other antiretroviral drugs. Their job is to target and block the reverse transcriptase enzyme, a critical tool the HIV virus needs to multiply.

Common NNRTIs:

- Delavirdine (Rescriptor)
- Efavirenz (Sustiva)
- Etravirine (Intelence)
- Nevirapine (Viramune)
- Rilpivirine (Edurant)

Pharmacokinetics: How the Body Handles Them

- Most NNRTIs (efavirenz, rilpivirine, etc.) are highly protein-bound and metabolized by liver enzymes—specifically the cytochrome P450 system.
- Nevirapine is widely distributed throughout the body.
- These drugs are cleared out via urine and feces.

Pharmacodynamics: How They Work

- Nevirapine and delavirdine physically bind to reverse transcriptase and block it.
- Efavirenz and rilpivirine work a bit differently—they compete with the enzyme using noncompetitive inhibition, essentially jamming the viral machine.

Pharmacotherapeutics: When They're Used

NNRTIs are always part of combination therapy for HIV.

- Nevirapine is often reserved for patients whose condition is worsening or whose immune function has significantly declined.

Drug Interactions to Know

- Nevirapine can lower the effectiveness of protease inhibitors and hormonal birth control—these shouldn't be used together.
- Delavirdine raises blood levels of several drugs (e.g., warfarin, benzodiazepines, saquinavir)—watch for toxicity.
- Efavirenz can reduce levels of indinavir and etravirine.
- Rilpivirine should NOT be combined with certain anticonvulsants, antimycobacterials, proton pump inhibitors, St. John's wort, or dexamethasone—these can reduce its effect and risk treatment failure.

Adverse Effects

Common side effects: headache, dizziness, nausea, vomiting, diarrhea, and weakness (asthenia).

Nevirapine can cause a severe, life-threatening rash. Discontinue if this occurs.

Nursing Process: NNRTIs

Assessment:

- Baseline and ongoing infection monitoring
- Check for drug interactions and side effects
- Assess patient/family understanding of treatment

Diagnoses:

- Risk for infection (hematologic side effects)
- Risk for fluid loss (from GI symptoms)
- Knowledge deficit

Goals:

- No injury or severe reactions
- Maintain hydration
- Patient/family understand medication plan

Implementation:

- Monitor renal, liver function, CBC, platelets
- Watch for CNS changes—safety precautions if needed
- Request antiemetics/antidiarrheals as needed
- Report serious reactions
- Educate about adherence and what to avoid

Evaluation:

- No adverse outcomes
- Stable hydration
- Patient/family can describe therapy and precautions

Nucleotide Reverse Transcriptase Inhibitors (NtRTIs)

NtRTIs are close cousins of the NRTIs—they also block reverse transcriptase but are built a bit differently at the molecular level.

Two Main Drugs in This Class:

- Tenofovir (Viread) – used for HIV
- Adefovir (Hepsera) – used for hepatitis B (HBV)

Pharmacokinetics:

Tenofovir is better absorbed with a high-fat meal; adefovir is not affected by food.

Both are minimally protein-bound and not metabolized by the P450 system.

Excreted mainly through the kidneys.

Pharmacodynamics:

- Tenofovir gets incorporated into the virus's DNA, stopping replication.
- Adefovir works the same way but is specific to HBV DNA.

Do not give adefovir and tenofovir together—they can interfere with each other.

Drug Interactions:

- Other kidney-eliminated drugs can raise tenofovir levels.
- Didanosine levels increase when used with tenofovir—monitor closely.

Adverse Reactions:

- Tenofovir: nausea, vomiting, diarrhea, anorexia, and abdominal pain.
- Adefovir: most common complaint is weakness.
- Both may cause life-threatening lactic acidosis and liver toxicity, especially in women, obese patients, or those on long-term therapy.

Nursing Process: NtRTIs

Assessment:

- Monitor viral load and side effects
- Review medications and interactions
- Assess for liver disease or risk factors

Diagnoses:

- Risk for hematologic side effects
- Risk for dehydration
- Deficient knowledge

Goals:

- Prevent complications
- Keep fluid balance
- Patient understands risks and usage

Implementation:

- Regular monitoring: renal, hepatic labs, CBC, electrolytes

- Watch for bone and fat distribution changes
- Educate about signs of lactic acidosis or liver issues
- Support with symptom relief (antiemetics, antidiarrheals)
- Take safety precautions for CNS side effects

Evaluation:

- Stable clinical status
- Hydration maintained
- Informed, engaged patient/family

Protease Inhibitors (PIs): Disrupting Viral Maturation

PIs stop HIV (and now HCV) from maturing by blocking the protease enzyme, which is essential for virus assembly. When blocked, new virus particles remain incomplete—and noninfectious.

Protease Inhibitors Include:

- Saquinavir (Invirase)
- Nelfinavir (Viracept)
- Ritonavir (Norvir)
- Indinavir (Crixivan)
- Lopinavir + Ritonavir (Kaletra)
- Fosamprenavir (Lexiva)
- Atazanavir (Reyataz)
- Darunavir (Prezista)
- Simeprevir, Tipranavir, Boceprevir – newer options, used for HIV or HCV

Pharmacokinetics:

- Many PIs are highly protein-bound and metabolized by the liver's cytochrome P450 system.
- Excretion is mostly via feces, with some renal clearance.

Some drugs (like lopinavir) are only available in combo with ritonavir, which boosts their blood levels by slowing metabolism.

Pharmacodynamics:

All PIs inhibit viral protease, preventing the virus from maturing into its infectious form.

Therapeutic Use:

- Combination HIV therapy
- HCV treatment with some newer agents

Drug Interactions:

These drugs have many interactions—especially with:

- CYP3A inhibitors/inducers
- Sedatives (midazolam, triazolam)
- Heart meds (amiodarone, diltiazem)
- Seizure meds (carbamazepine, phenytoin)
- Herbals like St. John's wort

Some combinations can lead to severe reactions—always check compatibility.

Adverse Effects:

Different PIs have different side effects. Here's a breakdown:

Saquinavir:

- Dizziness, increased lipids, body fat changes, GI upset, night sweats

Ritonavir:

- GI distress, altered taste, muscle pain

Indinavir:

- GI upset, fatigue, dry mouth, insomnia, back pain

Nelfinavir:

- Seizures, liver issues, hypoglycemia, allergic reactions

Fosamprenavir:

- Numbness, rash, nausea, diarrhea, hyperglycemia

Lopinavir + Ritonavir:

- Encephalopathy, blood clots, hemorrhagic colitis

Atazanavir:

- Heart rhythm changes, liver toxicity, lactic acidosis
- May prolong PR interval—use caution with heart meds

Simeprevir, Tipranavir, Boceprevir, Darunavir:

- Contain sulfa groups—avoid in sulfa allergies
- Common side effects: nausea, diarrhea, fatigue, rash

Nursing Process: Protease Inhibitors

Assessment:

- Baseline infection and labs
- Monitor drug interactions and effects
- Assess knowledge level

Diagnoses:

- Risk for injury
- Risk for dehydration
- Knowledge gap

Goals:

- Prevent complications
- Maintain hydration
- Ensure understanding of therapy

Implementation:

- Monitor renal, liver function, blood counts
- Check blood sugar in diabetic patients
- Administer with food as required
- Use CNS safety precautions as needed
- Educate on timing, interactions, and side effects
- Follow guidelines for prep/admin

Evaluation:

- No severe side effects
- Patient remains stable
- Family is confident and educated

HBV and HCV Antiviral Drugs: A Closer Look

The treatment of hepatitis B (HBV) and hepatitis C (HCV) involves several different drug classes, each working in its own unique way to control viral replication and support immune function. Here's what you need to know:

Drug Categories:

Biologic response modifiers:

- Interferon alfa-2b (Intron A)
- Interferon alfacon-1 (Infergen)

Nucleoside analogue:

- Entecavir (Baraclude)

Nucleotide analogue:

- Sofosbuvir (Sovaldi)

Virus proliferation inhibitors:

- Peginterferon alfa-2a (Pegasys)
- Peginterferon alfa-2b (PegIntron)

Pharmacokinetics: How These Drugs Move Through the Body

- Interferons and peginterferons: Not extensively studied; mostly broken down in the kidneys.
- Entecavir: Absorption is slowed by food, widely distributed in tissues, and mostly excreted unchanged by the kidneys.
- Sofosbuvir: Easily absorbed (food or no food), travels through plasma proteins, metabolized in the liver, excreted mostly in urine and some in feces.
- Peginterferons: Injected subcutaneously. Around 30% of alfa-2b is cleared by the kidneys.

Pharmacodynamics: How They Work

- Interferons: Bind to cell surface receptors and kick off a chain of immune responses that help suppress HBV replication.
- Entecavir: Mimics natural substances to block HBV gene transcription and replication.
- Sofosbuvir: A prodrug activated in the liver; once inside the viral RNA chain, it shuts down further replication.
- Peginterferons: These have "pleiotropic" effects—meaning they affect multiple systems. They suppress cell division and boost immune cell activity like phagocytosis.

Pharmacotherapeutics: What They're Used For

- Interferon alfacon-1: Used only for chronic HCV.
- Interferon alfa-2b: Used for both chronic HCV and HBV; also helps treat Kaposi's sarcoma (a cancer seen in some patients with AIDS).
- Entecavir: Treats only HBV.
- Sofosbuvir, peginterferon alfa-2a, and alfa-2b: Used in combination therapy for HCV. These are not effective alone.

Drug Interactions to Watch Out For

Interferons:

- Use cautiously with myelosuppressive drugs like zidovudine (watch for toxicity).
- Interferon alfa-2b raises theophylline levels—avoid combining them.
- All interferons and peginterferons are often combined with ribavirin, which they shouldn't be used with if the patient has a known sensitivity.

Entecavir:

- Since it's cleared through the kidneys, any drug affecting kidney function should be used cautiously.

Sofosbuvir:

- Don't give with rifampin, St. John's wort, or amiodarone (can cause serious bradycardia).
- Metabolized by P-glycoprotein—a lot of other meds affect this, including anticonvulsants, antimycobacterials, and HIV meds.

Peginterferons:

- Watch for increased toxicity when given with nucleoside analogues or methadone.
- Monitor closely when combined with zidovudine, especially for worsening anemia or neutropenia.

Pregnancy Warning

Many of these drugs—especially when combined with ribavirin—are highly toxic to developing fetuses.

Precautions include:

- Negative pregnancy test before starting treatment
- Monthly retesting

- Two forms of contraception (during therapy and for 6 months after)

Additional Warnings

Interferons and peginterferons carry boxed warnings for the risk of life-threatening:

- Neuropsychiatric effects (e.g., depression, suicidal thoughts)
- Autoimmune disorders
- Infections
- Ischemic events (e.g., heart attack or stroke)

Patients require regular, detailed clinical evaluations. If symptoms worsen, treatment may need to be stopped.

Common Adverse Reactions

- Flulike symptoms: headache, fever, fatigue, muscle aches, nausea
- Chills
- GI issues: abdominal pain
- Neutropenia (low white blood cell count)
- Injection site reactions

Nursing Process: HBV/HCV Therapy

Assessment:

- Baseline liver function, viral load, renal function
- Monitor for side effects and drug interactions
- Check understanding of drug safety (especially regarding pregnancy)

Diagnoses:

- Risk for infection due to immunosuppression
- Risk for dehydration from GI effects
- Knowledge deficit about medication

Goals:

- No injury or major side effects
- Stable hydration
- Clear understanding of therapy plan

Implementation:

- Monitor renal, liver labs, CBC, electrolytes
- Assess creatinine clearance frequently
- Watch for CNS changes, and ensure safety (bed rails, supervision)
- Administer meds per protocol
- Notify prescriber about serious or ongoing issues

Evaluation:

- Patient avoids complications
- Hydration maintained
- Patient and family understand the importance of adherence and safety

Antitubercular Drugs: Managing TB with Precision

Tuberculosis (TB) is caused by Mycobacterium tuberculosis and requires long-term, multi-drug therapy. This can make adherence and management a challenge—but it's critical for effective treatment and prevention of drug resistance.

Common TB Drugs (First-Line):

- Isoniazid (INH)
- Rifampin (RIF)
- Pyrazinamide (PZA)
- Ethambutol (EMB)

Often combined in formulations like Rifamate (isoniazid + rifampin) or Rifater (isoniazid + rifampin + pyrazinamide)

Treatment Duration & Challenges

TB meds may be needed for months.

Long-term therapy can lead to:

- Noncompliance
- Drug resistance
- Cumulative toxicity

If resistance is detected (e.g., to INH or RIF), 5- or 6-drug regimens may be needed—especially in institutional settings like hospitals or prisons.

Pharmacokinetics & Pharmacodynamics

- Absorption: Well absorbed orally
- Distribution: Widespread throughout body
- Metabolism: Mostly liver
- Excretion: Mainly kidneys

How they work:

- Isoniazid & ethambutol: Inhibit bacterial growth (tuberculostatic)
- Rifampin: Destroys mycobacteria (tuberculocidal)
- Pyrazinamide: Creates an acidic environment that halts TB replication

When They're Used

- Isoniazid: With others for active TB; alone for prophylaxis after exposure
- Ethambutol: For uncomplicated TB and other mycobacterial infections
- Rifampin: Used with other TB drugs; sometimes used to treat N. meningitidis carriers
- Pyrazinamide: First-line drug, always part of combination therapy

Drug Interactions

- INH increases levels of: phenytoin, theophylline, warfarin, etc.
- Rifampin can reduce effectiveness of birth control pills
- INH + corticosteroids: reduced INH effect, enhanced steroid effect
- Hepatotoxicity risk increases with combo use of INH, rifampin, pyrazinamide

Adverse Reactions

- Ethambutol: Vision problems (optic neuritis), joint pain, numbness, confusion
- Isoniazid: Peripheral neuropathy, hepatitis (can be fatal), rash
- Rifampin: GI upset, orange-colored body fluids, liver issues
- Pyrazinamide: Liver toxicity, nausea, vomiting, anorexia

Nursing Process: TB Treatment

Assessment:

- Initial culture and sensitivity
- Ongoing evaluation of effectiveness and side effects
- Educate patient and family

Diagnoses:

- Risk of infection
- Sensory changes (from neuropathy)
- Knowledge gap

Goals:

- TB is controlled (negative cultures, normal WBCs)
- Sensory symptoms are prevented
- Patient understands importance of adherence

Implementation:

- Give 1 hour before or 2 hours after meals

- Monitor for tingling or numbness
- Watch liver function and watch for jaundice
- Encourage follow-ups and adherence
- Educate about orange fluids (Rifampin) and side effects

Evaluation:

- Infection is under control
- No major sensory or hepatic complications
- Patient/family are informed and adherent

12.4. Antifungal drugs

Antifungal drugs—also known as antimycotics—are used to treat infections caused by fungi. These infections can range from mild, such as oral thrush or athlete's foot, to severe, life-threatening systemic infections. The major types of antifungals include:

- Polyenes
- Flucytosine
- Ketoconazole
- Synthetic triazoles
- Glucan synthesis inhibitors

Polyenes: Amphotericin B & Nystatin

Amphotericin B is one of the most powerful antifungals available and is often reserved for serious, systemic fungal infections. Nystatin, on the other hand, is only used topically or orally for localized fungal infections because it's too toxic to be given intravenously.

Pharmacokinetics

Amphotericin B is given by IV. It spreads throughout the body and is excreted by the kidneys. Its exact metabolic pathway isn't fully known.

Nystatin (oral) isn't absorbed into the bloodstream at all—it stays in the gut and is passed unchanged in the feces. Topical nystatin doesn't get absorbed through the skin or mucous membranes.

Pharmacodynamics

Amphotericin B works by binding to sterols in the fungal cell membrane, making the membrane "leaky" so vital cell contents spill out.

Nystatin works similarly and can either kill fungi (fungicidal) or just stop their growth (fungistatic), depending on the organism.

Pharmacotherapeutics

Amphotericin B is used to treat life-threatening fungal infections such as cryptococcal meningitis and infections caused by Candida, Aspergillus, and other rare fungi. It's not used for minor infections due to its high toxicity.

Nystatin is the go-to for:

- Oral thrush
- Diaper rash
- Vaginal yeast infections
- GI tract candidiasis (oral form)

Drug Interactions

Amphotericin B interacts with many drugs:

- Flucytosine + Amphotericin B = a powerful combination for tough infections.
- Increases risk of kidney damage when used with aminoglycosides or cyclosporine.
- Can worsen low potassium levels, which may increase the risk of heart problems.
- Can't be mixed with saline—must be diluted in D5W.

Nystatin doesn't significantly interact with other drugs.

Adverse Reactions

Most patients receiving IV amphotericin B experience:

- Fever, chills, nausea, vomiting

- Muscle or joint pain
- Loss of appetite
- Anemia (lower red blood cell count)
- Electrolyte imbalances (low potassium and magnesium)

Serious side effect: up to 80% may experience some degree of kidney toxicity.

High doses of nystatin may cause:

- GI distress
- Headaches
- Bitter taste
- Skin irritation (with topical use)
- Allergic reactions

Nursing Process for Polyenes

Assessment

- Get a full history and perform culture tests before starting.
- Monitor for side effects and potential interactions.
- Gauge patient/family knowledge about the medication.

Key Diagnoses

- Risk for infection due to underlying condition
- Risk for injury due to adverse reactions
- Lack of knowledge about drug therapy

Planning Goals

- Infection improves (based on labs and symptoms)
- No serious drug-related harm occurs
- Patient/family understands the medication plan

Implementation

- IV amphotericin B is for hospital use only and must be given slowly—never as a rapid infusion.

- Monitor vitals closely for the first few hours.
- Watch renal labs and electrolyte levels weekly (BUN, creatinine, potassium, magnesium).
- If serious side effects appear, stop the drug and notify the provider.
- Pre-medications (like antihistamines or antipyretics) may be ordered to reduce infusion reactions.

Evaluation

- Fungal infection resolves
- No injuries or complications from treatment
- Patient and family can explain the purpose and safety steps for therapy

Rewrite it and make it humanize. Do not skil so much content.

Ketoconazole is a synthetic imidazole derivative that's effective against a wide range of fungal infections. It's most often used for systemic or topical fungal infections and works by interfering with the fungus's ability to make essential sterols—components that keep its cell walls intact.

How the Body Handles Ketoconazole (Pharmacokinetics)

- When taken by mouth, ketoconazole is absorbed to varying degrees and spreads throughout the body.
- It's broken down in the liver and leaves the body mostly through bile and feces.

How It Works (Pharmacodynamics)

Once inside fungal cells, ketoconazole disrupts sterol production. This weakens the cell wall, makes it leaky, and ultimately stops the fungus from growing—or even kills it in some cases.

What It's Used For (Pharmacotherapeutics)

Ketoconazole is used for treating a range of fungal infections caused by susceptible fungi, including dermatophytes (which cause skin infections) and other fungi that cause systemic infections.

Drug Interactions: Things to Watch For

Ketoconazole can interact with many other medications

- It may increase levels of certain drugs like quinidine, sulfonylureas, carbamazepine, and HIV protease inhibitors.
- Rifampin can lower ketoconazole levels, making it less effective—so avoid this combo.
- Taking it with acid-reducing drugs (like antacids or H2-blockers) can reduce absorption. If needed, space them out by 2 hours.
- It can also interact with phenytoin, theophylline, cyclosporine, and oral anticoagulants, possibly increasing their levels or side effects.
- Combined use with other liver-toxic medications increases the risk of liver damage.

Adverse Reactions: What Might Happen

Common side effects include:

- Nausea and vomiting
- Rare but serious: anaphylaxis, hepatotoxicity, joint pain, chills, and photophobia
- May also cause tinnitus, sexual dysfunction (impotence), and reversible liver problems

Nursing Process: Caring for Patients on Ketoconazole

Assessment

- Check the type and severity of the fungal infection before starting treatment.
- Monitor for drug reactions and interactions.

- Assess the patient's and their family's understanding of the medication.

Key Nursing Diagnoses

- Risk for infection (due to underlying condition)
- Risk for fluid imbalance (from GI side effects)
- Lack of knowledge about medication

Planning Goals

- Infection resolves (as shown by culture, temperature, WBCs)
- No serious side effects occur
- Patient and family understand the treatment plan

Implementation Tips

- Don't use ketoconazole for minor infections like nail fungus or athlete's foot due to liver risks.
- Give with food to reduce nausea and divide doses if needed.
- Keep an eye on hydration and liver function.

Evaluation

- Infection clears
- Patient stays hydrated
- Patient and family are informed and confident in managing the therapy

Synthetic Triazoles: Modern Antifungal Options

These include fluconazole, itraconazole, voriconazole, and posaconazole. They're used to treat a range of serious fungal infections—and each comes with its own dosing quirks and drug interaction risks.

Pharmacokinetics (How They Move Through the Body)

- Fluconazole is well absorbed (90%) and mostly excreted unchanged in the urine.

- Itraconazole and posaconazole work best when taken with food, while voriconazole is more effective on an empty stomach.
- All are metabolized in the liver, with minimal fecal elimination.

How They Work (Pharmacodynamics)

- Fluconazole and posaconazole block fungal enzymes needed to build strong cell walls.
- Itraconazole and voriconazole disrupt the formation of ergosterol, a key fungal component, weakening the fungal cell and making it prone to destruction.

Therapeutic Uses

- Fluconazole: candidiasis of the mouth, throat, esophagus; systemic infections; cryptococcal meningitis
- Itraconazole: blastomycosis, histoplasmosis, fungal nail infections
- Voriconazole: invasive aspergillosis, infections from Scedosporium or Fusarium
- Posaconazole: prevention of fungal infections in high-risk patients (like transplant recipients); treatment of oropharyngeal candidiasis

Drug Interactions: The Big Ones

- Fluconazole can raise levels of warfarin, phenytoin, cyclosporine, and oral diabetes drugs, increasing side effects.
- Itraconazole and voriconazole have many interactions. They can increase bleeding risk with warfarin and interfere with a range of drugs (like phenytoin, benzodiazepines, sulfonylureas, and more).
- Voriconazole should never be used with sirolimus, ergot drugs, or certain heart medications due to risk of dangerous side effects like heart rhythm problems.

- Posaconazole affects a pathway called CYP3A4 and P-glycoprotein—so it can alter the levels of many other drugs. Monitor closely!

Adverse Reactions

Fluconazole, voriconazole, and posaconazole may cause:

- Headache, dizziness
- Nausea, vomiting, diarrhea
- Abdominal pain, rash
- Elevated liver enzymes

Itraconazole may cause:

- Dizziness, headache
- High blood pressure
- Liver issues
- Nausea

Nursing Process

Assessment

- Assess the type and severity of the infection
- Monitor liver function if treatment lasts a while
- Watch for drug interactions and adverse effects

Nursing Diagnoses

- Risk for infection
- Risk for dehydration
- Deficient knowledge

Goals

- Patient recovers from fungal infection
- Maintains hydration
- Demonstrates understanding of drug use

Implementation

- Handle IV forms carefully—don't open sterile packaging early
- Infuse fluconazole slowly (no more than 200 mg/hour)
- Avoid combining IV drugs in the same line
- If a rash occurs, monitor closely and notify the prescriber
- Keep an eye on hydration status during GI upset

Evaluation

- Patient recovers
- Stays hydrated
- Understands treatment plan

Glucan Synthesis Inhibitors: A Newer Approach

This group—also called echinocandins—includes:

- Caspofungin (Cancidas)
- Anidulafungin (Eraxis)
- Micafungin (Mycamine)

They're given by IV and used for serious fungal infections like candidemia and invasive aspergillosis.

How They Work

These drugs block beta-1,3-D-glucan, a component crucial for building the fungal cell wall. Without it, the fungus can't survive.

Who They're For

- Caspofungin: second-line for invasive aspergillosis
- Anidulafungin and micafungin: used for Candida infections and as fungal infection prevention in stem cell transplant patients

Drug Interactions

- Caspofungin can lower tacrolimus levels, so doses may need adjustment.

- Caspofungin + cyclosporine isn't a good combo—can raise liver enzymes and reduce clearance.
- Other enzyme inducers (like phenytoin, carbamazepine) can reduce caspofungin's effectiveness.

Adverse Reactions

Common across the group:

- Nausea, vomiting, diarrhea
- Fever

Caspofungin may also cause:

- Rash, tingling, fast heartbeat, fast breathing, facial swelling

Anidulafungin: insomnia, headache, indigestion, anemia

Micafungin: thrombocytopenia (low platelets), headache

Nursing Process

Assessment

- Check liver function before and during treatment
- Monitor for allergic-type reactions (facial swelling, itching, rash)
- Assess patient and family understanding

Nursing Diagnoses

- Risk for infection due to IV route
- Impaired health maintenance
- Knowledge deficit about therapy

Goals

- Infection clears
- Health maintained throughout therapy
- Patient and family are informed

Implementation

- Administer IV slowly over 1 hour

- Adjust doses for liver issues
- Monitor IV site for irritation or phlebitis
- Track liver enzymes regularly

Evaluation

- Infection resolves
- Treatment is well-tolerated
- Patient and family understand therapy plan

Chapter 13: Anti-Inflammatory, Antiallergy, and Immunosuppressant Medicines

13.1. Drugs and the Immune System

Your immune system and inflammatory response act as your body's built-in defense team, working constantly to protect you from harmful invaders like bacteria, viruses, and allergens. But sometimes, the immune response can go overboard—or it may need to be controlled, like after an organ transplant or during an autoimmune condition.

That's where certain drugs come in. These medications don't just fight off disease—they help regulate, calm, or redirect the immune system to maintain balance and prevent harm.

Here are some of the major classes of drugs that affect the immune and inflammatory responses:

Antihistamines

These drugs block the effects of histamine, a chemical the body releases during allergic reactions. Histamine is what causes symptoms like sneezing, itching, swelling, or hives.

By blocking histamine at its target sites (such as in the nose, skin, or lungs), antihistamines help reduce allergic symptoms and improve comfort during allergies, hay fever, or even insect bites.

Corticosteroids

Corticosteroids are powerful drugs that suppress the immune system and help reduce inflammation.

They're used in a wide range of conditions—from asthma and arthritis to autoimmune diseases like lupus. They work by mimicking your body's natural hormones (produced in the adrenal glands) to slow down or stop inflammatory processes that can damage tissue.

Immunosuppressants (Non-Corticosteroids)

These medications suppress or tone down the immune system—but without using corticosteroids.

They are especially important after organ transplants, helping the body avoid rejecting the new organ.

They're also useful in treating autoimmune conditions like rheumatoid arthritis, where the immune system mistakenly attacks healthy tissue.

Uricosurics

Uricosuric drugs help prevent gout attacks by controlling the level of uric acid in the body.

When uric acid builds up in the blood, it can form crystals in the joints, causing painful inflammation (gouty arthritis). These drugs help the kidneys remove excess uric acid through the urine, lowering the risk of flare-ups.

13.2. Antihistamines

Antihistamines are best known as go-to medications for allergies—they help calm the body's reaction to things like pollen, dust, or pet dander. Specifically, they block the effects of histamine, a chemical released during an immediate (type I) hypersensitivity reaction, also known as an allergic response.

They're widely available—some are prescription-only, while many can be found over the counter, either as standalone drugs or in combination with other medications.

How They Work: H1-Receptor Antagonists

Most antihistamines target histamine-1 (H1) receptors. These drugs compete with histamine for these receptors throughout the body, but they don't kick off any histamine that's already attached. Instead, they work to prevent histamine from binding in the first place, reducing or stopping the allergic response.

Classes of Antihistamines (By Chemical Structure)

Antihistamines come in several categories, grouped by their chemistry:

- Ethanolamines: clemastine fumarate, dimenhydrinate, diphenhydramine
- Alkylamines: brompheniramine, chlorpheniramine, dexchlorpheniramine
- Phenothiazines: promethazine
- Piperidines: azatadine, cetirizine, cyproheptadine, desloratadine, fexofenadine, loratadine, meclizine
- Miscellaneous: hydroxyzine hydrochloride, hydroxyzine pamoate

How the Body Handles Them (Pharmacokinetics)

Most H1-receptor antagonists are well absorbed after being taken orally or by injection, and some can also be given rectally. Once absorbed, they're widely distributed, including into the central nervous system (CNS)—which is why many cause drowsiness.

However, nonsedating antihistamines like fexofenadine, loratadine, and desloratadine don't easily cross the blood-brain barrier, so they have fewer sedative effects.

These drugs are broken down in the liver and mostly eliminated in the urine, though fexofenadine is mostly excreted in feces.

How They Act (Pharmacodynamics)

By blocking H1 receptors, these drugs prevent histamine from doing its job—which is a good thing during an allergic reaction. They help by:

- Reducing blood vessel dilation and tissue swelling
- Decreasing leaky capillaries that cause edema
- Blocking bronchial and gastrointestinal smooth muscle contractions

- Calming the itching and redness caused by histamine in the skin
- Suppressing some autonomic nervous system responses, such as watery eyes or salivation

Some antihistamines, like diphenhydramine and promethazine, cross into the brain and are used for their sedative or anti-nausea effects.

Note: H1 antihistamines don't affect stomach acid secretion. That's controlled by H2 receptors, which are blocked by a different class of drugs.

What They're Used For (Pharmacotherapeutics)

Antihistamines help manage symptoms of allergic reactions, including:

- Allergic rhinitis (runny nose, itchy eyes)
- Vasomotor rhinitis (non-allergic nasal irritation)
- Allergic conjunctivitis (eye inflammation)
- Urticaria (hives)
- Angioedema (swelling in the face, hands, or feet)

But that's not all—they're also used for:

- Nausea and vomiting (especially motion sickness)
- Anaphylaxis (as supportive therapy after epinephrine)
- Parkinson's disease symptoms and drug-induced movement disorders
- Serotonin-related conditions, like Cushing's disease or cluster headaches (cyproheptadine)

Watch Out for Drug Interactions

Antihistamines can interact with other drugs in potentially serious ways:

- They may block or reverse the effects of epinephrine, lowering blood pressure and increasing heart rate.
- They can mask signs of ear toxicity caused by some antibiotics or high-dose aspirin.
- They increase sedation when combined with alcohol, tranquilizers, or other CNS depressants.

- Loratadine can cause dangerous heart effects if taken with certain antibiotics or antifungals (like erythromycin or ketoconazole).

Possible Side Effects

The most common issue—especially with older antihistamines—is CNS depression (think drowsiness or grogginess). Other side effects can include:

Nervous system:

- Dizziness
- Fatigue
- Muscle weakness
- Poor coordination

Digestive system:

- Nausea, vomiting, constipation, or diarrhea
- Loss of appetite
- Dry mouth, nose, or throat

Heart and blood vessels:

- Low or high blood pressure
- Fast or irregular heartbeats

Other:

- Allergic reactions in sensitive individuals
- Nursing Process for Antihistamines

Assessment

- Review the patient's history and current condition.
- Monitor for side effects and possible drug interactions.
- For long-term use, check blood work for any signs of blood disorders.
- Assess the patient's and family's understanding of the medication.

Key Nursing Diagnoses

- Ineffective health maintenance
- Risk for injury due to sedation or dizziness
- Knowledge deficit about the medication

Planning Goals

- The patient shows improvement in symptoms.
- The patient remains safe and injury-free.
- The patient and family understand how to take the medication properly.

Implementation

- Give with food to reduce stomach upset.
- Follow IV administration guidelines carefully.
- For IM injections, rotate sites and inject into large muscles.
- Offer sugar-free gum or ice chips for dry mouth.
- Encourage fluids or use a humidifier if secretions are thick.
- Let the provider know if the drug stops being effective—an alternative may be needed.

Evaluation

- The patient has symptom relief.
- No injuries or complications occur from the drug.
- The patient and family can explain how and why the drug is used.

13.3. Corticosteroids

Corticosteroids are powerful medications that suppress the immune system and reduce inflammation. They're either naturally produced by the adrenal glands or synthesized in labs to mimic the body's natural hormones.

A Look at the Types

Your adrenal cortex makes two main types of corticosteroids:

- Glucocorticoids (like cortisone and dexamethasone) help manage how your body processes carbs, fats, and proteins.
- Mineralocorticoids (like aldosterone and fludrocortisone) help regulate electrolytes and water balance in the body.

Most of the corticosteroid medications you'll come across are synthetic versions of these natural hormones.

Glucocorticoids: Multi-Purpose Workhorses

These drugs are widely used due to their anti-inflammatory, immunosuppressant, and metabolic effects. Common examples include:

- beclomethasone
- betamethasone
- cortisone
- dexamethasone
- hydrocortisone
- methylprednisolone
- prednisolone
- prednisone
- triamcinolone

How They Move Through the Body (Pharmacokinetics)

Glucocorticoids are well absorbed when taken by mouth or injected into muscle. They travel through the bloodstream bound to plasma proteins, are broken down in the liver, and eliminated via the kidneys.

How They Work (Pharmacodynamics)

Although the exact process isn't fully understood, glucocorticoids are believed to:

- Suppress cell-mediated immune responses
- Lower white blood cell counts, especially leukocytes, monocytes, and eosinophils
- Reduce the binding of antibodies to cell receptors
- Inhibit interleukin production

On the inflammatory side, they:

- Stabilize lysosomal membranes, preventing the release of damaging enzymes
- Reduce capillary leakage, swelling, and redness
- Suppress immune cell movement to injury sites and limit phagocytosis
- Inhibit histamine production, collagen development, capillary dilation, and permeability

What They're Used For (Pharmacotherapeutics)

Glucocorticoids are used to:

- Replace hormones in adrenocortical insufficiency
- Suppress immune responses (e.g., in allergies, autoimmune conditions)
- Treat inflammatory disorders like arthritis
- Manage certain blood and lymphatic diseases

Drug Interactions to Know

Some drugs may reduce or amplify glucocorticoid effects:

- Reduced effect: barbiturates, phenytoin, rifampin
- Increased potassium loss: with diuretics like furosemide or amphotericin B
- Increased glucocorticoid effect: with erythromycin or oral estrogen
- Decreased vaccine effectiveness
- Increased risk of ulcers when taken with NSAIDs or salicylates
- Worsened blood sugar control when taken with antidiabetic drugs

Side Effects to Watch For

Because they act systemically, glucocorticoids can affect nearly every part of the body, especially when used long-term or at high doses. Possible adverse effects include:

General:

- Insomnia
- Personality changes
- Increased infection risk

Fluid & Electrolyte Imbalance:

- Sodium and water retention
- Potassium loss

Serious Concerns:

- Osteoporosis
- Peptic ulcers
- Delayed wound healing
- Cataracts
- Hypertension
- Intestinal perforation

Endocrine Effects:

- High blood sugar
- Adrenal gland shrinkage
- Cushingoid symptoms (e.g., moon face, buffalo hump)

Nursing Process for Glucocorticoids

Assessment

- Check patient's condition and establish baselines (BP, weight, electrolytes).
- Watch closely for depression, psychosis, or blood sugar changes.
- Monitor for signs of infection.
- Assess understanding of the medication.
- Monitor children for growth delays.

Key Nursing Diagnoses

- Disturbed body image from physical changes
- Risk for infection due to immune suppression
- Lack of knowledge about medication use

Planning Goals

- Prevent serious side effects
- Keep patient free from infection
- Ensure understanding of therapy by patient and family

Implementation

- Give doses early in the day to follow natural hormone rhythms.
- Administer with food to reduce stomach upset.
- Increase dose during stress (e.g., illness, surgery).
- Never stop abruptly—tapering is essential.
- Watch for and report serious side effects.
- Provide low-sodium, high-potassium, high-protein diet if allowed.
- Potassium supplements may be necessary.

Evaluation

- Patient shows no signs of adrenal insufficiency.
- Patient avoids infection.
- Patient and family understand how to manage therapy.

Mineralocorticoids: Maintaining Balance

One main mineralocorticoid used clinically is fludrocortisone acetate, a synthetic version of aldosterone.

How It Works

Fludrocortisone helps the body retain sodium and water and excrete potassium and hydrogen, which is crucial for fluid balance and blood pressure regulation.

When It's Used

- As replacement therapy in adrenocortical insufficiency
- In salt-losing conditions, like congenital adrenal hyperplasia (once electrolyte balance is restored)

Pharmacokinetics

This drug is well absorbed, spreads throughout the body, is broken down in the liver, and excreted by the kidneys.

Drug Interactions & Adverse Reactions

Mineralocorticoids share many interactions and side effects with glucocorticoids, especially related to electrolyte imbalances, fluid retention, and blood pressure changes.

Nursing Process for Mineralocorticoids

Assessment

- Check BP, weight, and electrolytes before and during therapy.
- Monitor closely for adverse reactions.
- Ensure patient and family understand the medication.

Key Nursing Diagnoses

- Risk for injury due to side effects
- Deficient fluid volume from poor drug response
- Lack of knowledge about therapy

Planning Goals

- Patient avoids serious side effects
- Patient maintains healthy fluid and electrolyte levels
- Patient and family understand how and why to take the medication

Implementation

- Follow dosage instructions carefully.

- Report any signs of hypertension or hypokalemia (muscle cramps, EKG changes).
- Potassium supplements may be needed.

Evaluation

- Patient has no adverse reactions
- Fluid, sodium, and potassium levels remain stable
- Patient and family understand how to manage therapy

13.4. Immunosuppressants

Immunosuppressants are powerful medications used to tone down the immune system, especially in patients who have received organ transplants. They help prevent the body from rejecting a new organ (a process called allograft rejection). Some of these drugs are also used—sometimes experimentally—to treat autoimmune diseases, where the body mistakenly attacks itself.

Here are some of the key players in this drug class:

- Anakinra
- Azathioprine
- Basiliximab
- Cyclosporine
- Daclizumab
- Lymphocyte immune globulin (ATG [equine])
- Muromonab-CD3
- Mycophenolate mofetil
- Sirolimus
- Tacrolimus
- Thymoglobulin (antithymocyte globulin [rabbit])

How these drugs travel through the body (Pharmacokinetics)

Each of these immunosuppressants takes its own route through the body:

- Azathioprine is quickly absorbed when taken orally. In contrast, cyclosporine and sirolimus are absorbed more slowly and not as completely.
- IV-only drugs include ATG, muromonab-CD3, anakinra, basiliximab, daclizumab, and thymoglobulin.
- Cyclosporine and muromonab-CD3 are known to spread widely in the body. Azathioprine and cyclosporine also cross the placenta.
- Most of these drugs are broken down in the liver and exit the body through urine, bile, or feces—though each drug varies.

How they work (Pharmacodynamics)

Not all mechanisms are fully understood, but here's what we know:

- Azathioprine interferes with DNA and RNA production, slowing down immune cell activity.
- Cyclosporine seems to target helper and suppressor T cells, preventing them from overreacting.
- ATG may eliminate or alter T cells directly.
- Muromonab-CD3 blocks T-cell activity, while mycophenolate suppresses both T and B cells, limiting antibody production and inflammation.
- Sirolimus prevents T-cell activation and proliferation.
- Anakinra, basiliximab, and daclizumab all block interleukin activity—key messengers in the immune response.

When they're used (Pharmacotherapeutics)

The main role of these drugs is to prevent organ rejection in transplant patients. However, some are being explored or used to treat autoimmune disorders. For example:

- Cyclophosphamide, though primarily a cancer drug, has immunosuppressant uses.
- Anakinra is used in moderate to severe rheumatoid arthritis, especially when other treatments haven't worked.

What to watch for: Drug interactions

Immunosuppressants don't always play nice with other drugs. Some key interactions include:

- Allopurinol can raise azathioprine levels.
- Verapamil boosts sirolimus levels.
- Cyclosporine levels increase with antifungals, antibiotics, and hormonal contraceptives.
- Mycophenolate may be less effective when taken with antacids or cholestyramine.
- Kidney toxicity is more likely if cyclosporine is combined with drugs like acyclovir or aminoglycosides.
- Immunosuppressants + other immunosuppressants = higher risk of infection and lymphoma.
- Tacrolimus and sirolimus levels may be affected by enzyme inducers or inhibitors.

Side effects to be aware of (Adverse reactions)

Unfortunately, these drugs can cause significant side effects:

Azathioprine

- Bone marrow suppression
- Liver toxicity
- Nausea/vomiting

Cyclosporine

- Kidney and liver damage
- High potassium levels
- Infection risk

Daclizumab

- GI issues
- Chest pain, breathing problems
- Hypertension or hypotension

ATG and Thymoglobulin

- Fever, chills
- Low WBCs or platelets
- Headache, abdominal pain, systemic infection

Muromonab-CD3

- Tremors, fever
- Pulmonary edema
- Nausea/vomiting

Mycophenolate

- GI upset
- Leukopenia
- Liver enzyme changes
- Skin rash

Sirolimus

- Tremors
- Anemia
- Muscle/joint pain
- High cholesterol

Tacrolimus

- Nephrotoxicity
- Hypertension
- GI symptoms
- Hepatotoxicity

Nursing process in action

Assessment

Evaluate immune status and organ function.

Monitor for signs of rejection and infection.

Check labs: CBC, liver and kidney function, WBCs, platelets, and electrolytes.

Key nursing diagnoses

- Ineffective protection (risk of organ rejection)
- Risk for infection
- Deficient knowledge of therapy

Planning

- Maintain stable vital signs and labs.
- Prevent infection and organ rejection.
- Educate patient and family thoroughly.

Implementation

- Administer drugs exactly as prescribed.
- Monitor closely for fever, sore throat, or malaise.
- Avoid IM injections if platelets are low.
- Educate women on pregnancy risks during and after therapy.
- Remind patients it may take up to 12 weeks for full therapeutic effect.

Evaluation

- No signs of organ rejection.
- No serious infections.
- Patient and family understand the purpose and precautions of drug therapy.

13.5. Uricosurics and Other Antigout Drug

Uricosurics and antigout medications work by targeting uric acid, which plays a central role in gout—a painful form of arthritis. Gout flares up when uric acid builds up in the blood (a condition called hyperuricemia) and forms needle-like crystals in the joints, causing swelling, redness, and pain. This buildup can happen because the body either produces too much uric acid or doesn't get rid of enough through the kidneys.

Uricosuric Drugs: Pushing Uric Acid Out

The two main uricosuric drugs are probenecid and sulfinpyrazone, both of which increase uric acid excretion through the urine. These medications help manage and prevent gout attacks, but they aren't used during an active flare-up because they can worsen inflammation if started at the wrong time.

Pharmacokinetics (How They Move Through the Body)

- These drugs are well absorbed from the GI tract.
- They bind strongly to plasma proteins—up to 95% for probenecid and 98% for sulfinpyrazone.
- They're metabolized in the liver and primarily excreted by the kidneys.

Pharmacodynamics (How They Work)

Probenecid and sulfinpyrazone reduce how much uric acid is reabsorbed by the kidneys. Instead of being recycled, more uric acid is flushed out in urine—leading to lower levels in the blood.

Uses

- Treating chronic gout symptoms and preventing flare-ups
- Managing gouty arthritis (inflammation in joints caused by uric acid crystals)
- Addressing tophaceous gout (uric acid crystal deposits under the skin)
- Probenecid is also used to help the body eliminate excess uric acid in cases of persistent hyperuricemia.

Important Note: Don't start these drugs during a gout attack. They could make the flare worse. To reduce the risk of an attack when starting therapy, colchicine is often prescribed for the first 3 to 6 months as a preventative measure.

Drug Interactions

These drugs interact with a wide variety of medications:

- Probenecid can boost and prolong the effects of penicillins, sulfonamides, and cephalosporins.
- It can increase blood levels of methotrexate, dapsone, and aminosalicylic acid, raising the risk of toxicity.
- Sulfinpyrazone enhances the effects of warfarin, increasing the bleeding risk.
- Aspirin and other salicylates reduce sulfinpyrazone's effectiveness.
- Sulfinpyrazone can amplify the effects of oral antidiabetic medications, potentially leading to low blood sugar.

Adverse Reactions

- Common to both: Uric acid stones and blood-related issues
- Probenecid: Nausea, vomiting, headache, loss of appetite, and hypersensitivity
- Sulfinpyrazone: GI upset, indigestion, stomach pain, and potential bleeding

Nursing Process

Assessment

- Monitor kidney function (especially in long-term therapy); the drug isn't effective in patients with chronic kidney issues (GFR <30 mL/min).
- Watch for signs of GI upset or other side effects.
- Review the patient's knowledge of their medication and encourage questions.

Key Diagnoses

- Risk for dehydration or GI discomfort
- Ineffective health maintenance due to lack of knowledge

Planning Goals

- The patient stays well-hydrated and experiences fewer or no gout flares.

- The patient and family understand the purpose and proper use of medication.

Implementation

- Give medications with food, milk, or antacids to reduce GI side effects.
- Encourage plenty of fluids (at least 2 liters/day) to prevent uric acid kidney stones.
- Avoid alcohol and high-purine foods like sardines, liver, and anchovies.
- Start therapy only after the acute attack has subsided.
- Aspirin should be avoided—it may reduce the effectiveness of treatment.
- Let the prescriber know if symptoms worsen, or if any new side effects occur.

Other Antigout Drugs

Allopurinol and colchicine are also used to treat gout but work differently:

- Allopurinol blocks the production of uric acid by inhibiting the enzyme xanthine oxidase.
- Colchicine helps reduce inflammation by stopping white blood cells from attacking uric acid crystals in the joints.

Pharmacokinetics

- Allopurinol is absorbed in the GI tract, metabolized by the liver, and excreted in urine.
- Colchicine is absorbed, re-circulated through the liver and intestines, and primarily excreted in feces.

Pharmacotherapeutics

Allopurinol is used to:

- Prevent gouty attacks

- Treat high uric acid during cancer treatment
- Prevent kidney stones caused by uric acid

Colchicine is most effective at relieving pain during an acute gout flare and is often used with other meds like allopurinol early in therapy.

Drug Interactions

Allopurinol can increase the effects of:

- Oral anticoagulants
- Mercaptopurine, azathioprine (raising toxicity risk)
- Theophylline

It may also increase the risk of allergic reactions with ACE inhibitors.

Colchicine doesn't have major interactions but should be used cautiously in combination therapy.

Adverse Reactions

- Both can cause nausea, vomiting, diarrhea, and abdominal discomfort.
- Allopurinol may cause rashes—often the first sign of a serious allergic reaction. Stop the drug immediately if one appears.
- Colchicine, when used long-term, may lead to bone marrow suppression.

Nursing Process

Assessment

- Monitor uric acid levels and signs of gout or kidney issues.
- Regularly check liver and kidney function, as well as CBC.

Implementation

- Administer with meals to reduce GI upset.
- Encourage hydration to help flush uric acid.
- Use caution in patients with impaired kidney function.

- Educate patients to recognize and report side effects, especially rash or signs of infection.
- Remind patients that alcohol raises uric acid levels—avoid it during therapy.

Evaluation

- The patient has fewer or no gout attacks.
- No signs of infection or serious side effects.
- The patient and family understand how to manage gout and the purpose of their medications.

Chapter 14: Antineoplastic Medicines

14.1. Drugs and cancer

Back in the 1940s, the first antineoplastic drugs—also known as chemotherapy agents—were developed to help fight cancer. These early treatments marked a major medical breakthrough, but they often came with harsh side effects that took a heavy toll on patients.

A Shift for the Better

Thankfully, cancer treatment has come a long way. Today's chemotherapeutic drugs are generally less toxic, meaning patients don't suffer as much from the side effects that once made treatment incredibly difficult. With modern therapies, many cancers that were once fatal are now treatable—and even curable. For example:

- Acute lymphoblastic leukemia in children
- Testicular cancer in adults

These are now considered highly curable with appropriate treatment.

Newer approaches are also changing the game. Monoclonal antibodies and targeted therapies—which zero in on specific proteins or cancer-related mechanisms—are helping to extend remission periods and improve outcomes. In some cases, the body's own immune system can be used as part of the treatment plan. Interferons, for example, are being used in certain cancers to help fight tumor cells by boosting immune response.

Types of Antineoplastic Agents

There's now a wide range of cancer-fighting drugs, each working in a different way. These include:

- Alkylating agents – damage DNA to prevent cancer cells from reproducing
- Antimetabolites – disrupt cancer cell metabolism
- Antineoplastic antibiotics – interfere with cancer cell DNA replication
- Hormonal therapies and hormone modulators – slow cancers that rely on hormones to grow
- Natural products – derived from plants or microbes, they can interfere with cell division
- Monoclonal antibodies – target specific markers on cancer cells
- Topoisomerase I inhibitors – block enzymes involved in DNA repair
- Targeted therapies – act on specific proteins or genes involved in cancer growth
- Unclassified antineoplastics – drugs that don't fit into the traditional categories but still help fight cancer

14.2. Alkylating drugs

Alkylating drugs are a cornerstone of cancer treatment. Whether used alone or in combination with other therapies, these powerful medications target a wide range of cancers by interfering with DNA—ultimately stopping cancer cells from growing and multiplying.

These drugs fall into six main categories:

- Nitrogen mustards
- Alkyl sulfonates
- Nitrosoureas
- Triazines
- Ethylenimines
- Alkylating-like drugs

How They Work: Any Time, Any Phase

Alkylating agents attack the cancer cell's DNA, forming chemical bonds (called cross-links) that prevent the DNA strands from aligning properly. This disrupts replication and leads to cell death. What makes these drugs especially powerful is that they are not phase-specific—they can work at any stage of the cell cycle.

Nitrogen Mustards

This is the largest and most well-known group of alkylating agents. Common drugs include:

- Chlorambucil
- Cyclophosphamide
- Estramustine
- Ifosfamide
- Mechlorethamine hydrochloride
- Melphalan

Fun fact: Mechlorethamine was the first nitrogen mustard developed for cancer treatment—and it works fast.

Pharmacokinetics (How the Body Handles These Drugs)

Nitrogen mustards vary in how they're absorbed and distributed. Most are processed in the liver and eliminated through the kidneys. Mechlorethamine, for instance, is metabolized so quickly that within minutes, no active drug remains in the body.

Pharmacodynamics (How the Drugs Work)

These drugs form covalent bonds with DNA, disrupting its structure and function. But cancer cells can sometimes develop resistance, reducing drug effectiveness over time.

Therapeutic Uses

Nitrogen mustards are especially effective in treating cancers that involve elevated or abnormal white blood cell (WBC) activity, such as:

- Hodgkin's disease
- Leukemia

- Lymphomas
- Multiple myeloma
- Melanoma

They're also used to treat cancers of the breast, ovaries, uterus, brain, lungs, prostate, bladder, stomach, and testes.

Drug Interactions

These drugs can interact with many others:

- Estramustine: Absorption is reduced by calcium-rich foods or antacids.
- Cyclophosphamide: Increases cardiac risk if used with cardiotoxic drugs; can reduce digoxin levels.
- Ifosfamide: Risk of toxicity rises with allopurinol, barbiturates, phenytoin, or chloral hydrate.
- Melphalan: Its effects may be altered by corticosteroids or interferon alfa; combining with carmustine may increase lung toxicity.

Adverse Effects

- Fatigue is common
- Bone marrow suppression, which may lead to low WBCs (leukopenia) and platelets (thrombocytopenia)
- Nausea and vomiting due to CNS effects
- Stomatitis (inflammation in the mouth)
- Reversible hair loss

Safety Note: These drugs are vesicants, meaning they can cause severe skin and tissue damage if they leak outside the vein or come into contact with the skin, eyes, or respiratory tract.

Nursing Process: Nitrogen Mustards

Assessment

- Perform a complete physical assessment before and during therapy

- Monitor lab values: CBC, WBC, platelets, liver enzymes, kidney function, uric acid
- Check vital signs and IV/catheter sites regularly
- Watch closely for adverse effects or drug interactions
- Assess the patient's and family's understanding of the treatment

Nursing Diagnoses

- Ineffective health maintenance (due to cancer)
- Ineffective protection (due to reduced immune response)
- Deficient knowledge (regarding therapy)

Planning Goals

- Patient shows improvement in cancer symptoms and lab markers
- No signs of infection or bleeding
- Patient and caregivers understand the purpose and safety of therapy

Implementation

- Handle and dispose of chemotherapy drugs safely
- Keep emergency meds (like epinephrine, antihistamines, corticosteroids) on hand in case of allergic reactions
- Administer antiemetics for nausea
- Encourage hydration and monitor fluid balance
- Use strict infection control if WBC < 2,000/μL or granulocytes < 1,000/μL

Evaluation

- Cancer is controlled or improving on follow-up tests
- No infection or unusual bleeding
- Patient and caregivers can verbalize understanding of treatment

Alkyl Sulfonates: Busulfan

Busulfan is typically used to treat:

- Chronic myelogenous leukemia (CML)
- Polycythemia vera
- Other bone marrow disorders

It's also used in high doses before bone marrow transplants.

How It Works

Busulfan disrupts DNA by forming covalent bonds—similar to nitrogen mustards. It targets granulocytes (a type of WBC) and, to a lesser degree, platelets.

Pharmacokinetics

- Absorbed well from the GI tract
- Metabolized in the liver
- Half-life is around 2–3 hours
- Eliminated through the urine

Adverse Reactions

- Myelosuppression (severe drop in WBCs, RBCs, and platelets)
- Pulmonary fibrosis – may appear months to years after treatment
- Seizures – may occur in high doses

Drug Interactions

- Increases bleeding risk with aspirin or anticoagulants
- Use with thioguanine may lead to liver toxicity or portal hypertension
- Use with metronidazole may raise busulfan levels, increasing toxicity risk

Nursing Process: Busulfan

Assessment

- Monitor WBC and platelets weekly

- Watch for signs of improvement (e.g., increased appetite, smaller spleen)
- Monitor uric acid levels and assess for signs of toxicity

Implementation

- Give at the same time daily
- Adjust dose based on blood counts
- Often combined with allopurinol and hydration to prevent uric acid buildup
- Stop breastfeeding during treatment due to toxicity risk

Evaluation

- Patient responds positively to treatment
- No signs of infection
- Patient and family understand the treatment plan

Nitrosoureas: Brain-Savvy Fighters

Nitrosoureas include:

- Carmustine
- Lomustine
- Streptozocin

These drugs are fat-soluble, meaning they can cross the blood-brain barrier—a major advantage in treating brain tumors and meningeal leukemias.

How They Work

Through bifunctional alkylation, these agents interfere with DNA and proteins needed for cancer cells to divide.

Pharmacokinetics

- Carmustine (IV) and lomustine (oral) are well distributed in body tissues and CSF
- Streptozocin is only given IV (poor oral absorption)

- All are metabolized extensively and excreted in urine

Drug Interactions

- Cimetidine may increase bone marrow toxicity with carmustine
- Lomustine + anticoagulants or aspirin = increased bleeding risk
- Streptozocin may prolong effects of doxorubicin, worsening bone marrow suppression

Adverse Reactions

- Severe nausea and vomiting
- Bone marrow suppression (delayed onset: 4–6 weeks post-treatment)
- Kidney toxicity, possibly leading to kidney failure
- Reversible liver toxicity with high-dose carmustine
- Delayed pulmonary toxicity with carmustine—can occur up to 15 years later

Nursing Process: Nitrosoureas

Assessment

- Obtain baseline pulmonary function tests
- Regularly monitor CBC, liver, kidney, and lung function
- Check for adverse reactions and drug interactions
- Ensure patient and caregivers understand the therapy

Implementation

- Give antiemetics before treatment
- Follow safety protocols for handling and administration
- Use glass containers for carmustine (unstable in plastic)
- Avoid skin contact—can stain or cause damage

Evaluation

- Disease shows improvement
- Patient avoids major complications or toxicities

- Patient and family feel confident and informed about treatment

Double, Double, Avoid That Trouble... (Safety Measures During Chemotherapy).

Some chemotherapy drugs, like carmustine, need extra care during handling and administration:

- Always wear double gloves when handling carmustine wafers in the operating room to prevent skin exposure.
- Provide adequate hydration and monitor the patient's fluid intake and output—this helps protect the kidneys from toxicity.
- Allopurinol may be prescribed alongside hydration to prevent high uric acid levels and potential kidney complications.
- If the patient is breastfeeding, advise them to stop during therapy due to the risk of passing the drug to the infant.
- Only repeat lomustine doses when the CBC (complete blood count) shows that blood cell levels have safely recovered.
- Implement strict infection prevention and bleeding precautions, especially in patients with low white cell or platelet counts.

Evaluation:

- The patient shows improvement in their cancer based on follow-up tests.
- No injuries or complications occur due to adverse drug effects.
- The patient and their family understand the therapy plan and what to watch for.

Triazines: Dacarbazine

Dacarbazine is a triazine drug that becomes active only after it's metabolized by the liver. It's primarily used to treat malignant melanoma and is often combined with other drugs for Hodgkin's disease.

How It Works

Once activated, dacarbazine interferes with RNA and protein synthesis, halting cancer cell growth. Like other alkylating agents, it's cell cycle–nonspecific, meaning it works regardless of where the cancer cell is in its growth cycle.

Pharmacokinetics

- Given IV and distributed throughout the body
- Metabolized in the liver
- Excreted mainly through the kidneys (some unchanged, some as metabolites)
- Patients with liver or kidney dysfunction may have a longer drug half-life—up to 7 hours

Adverse Effects

- Low WBCs and platelets (leukopenia, thrombocytopenia)
- Nausea and vomiting (usually within 1–3 hours of treatment, lasting up to 12 hours)
- Hair loss
- Phototoxicity (sensitivity to sunlight)
- Flu-like syndrome (may occur about a week after treatment and last 1–3 weeks)

Nursing Process

Assessment

- Assess the patient's cancer type and treatment response regularly
- Monitor CBC, kidney, and liver function
- Evaluate IV site patency, vital signs, and watch for adverse effects

Diagnoses

- Ineffective health maintenance

- Risk for injury (from adverse effects)
- Deficient knowledge

Planning Goals

- Patient's cancer improves as shown by labs/imaging
- No signs of infection or excessive bleeding
- Patient and family understand the treatment and side effects

Implementation

- Handle and dispose of dacarbazine safely
- Give antiemetics before treatment to help with nausea
- Protect the IV bag from sunlight during infusion
- If the drug turns pink, discard it—it's no longer stable
- Avoid extravasation; if it occurs, stop the infusion, apply ice, and notify the prescriber
- Advise the patient to avoid sun exposure for 2 days after treatment
- Treat flu-like symptoms with acetaminophen (not aspirin)

Evaluation

- Patient improves based on follow-up results
- No infections or bleeding complications occur
- Patient and caregiver demonstrate understanding

Ethylenimines: Thiotepa

Thiotepa is a multifunctional alkylating drug used for:

- Bladder cancer
- Ovarian and breast carcinomas
- Lymphomas
- Treating intracavitary effusions (fluid build-up in chest or abdomen)
- Sometimes used in lung cancer

How It Works

Thiotepa interferes with DNA and RNA, preventing cell replication and leading to cell death. It crosses the blood-brain barrier and is excreted in the urine.

Adverse Effects

- Blood-related: pancytopenia, leukopenia, anemia, thrombocytopenia
- Nausea, vomiting, stomatitis, and mucosal ulceration
- Occasional rash, hives, and itching

GI symptoms may reverse in 6–8 months after stopping therapy.

Drug Interactions

- May increase bleeding risk if taken with aspirin or anticoagulants
- May prolong muscle paralysis when taken with neuromuscular blockers
- Can increase toxicity when used with other chemo or radiation
- May cause respiratory depression when combined with succinylcholine

Nursing Process

Assessment

- Monitor CBC weekly for 3 weeks after last dose
- Track uric acid levels, vital signs, and IV site
- Assess for any signs of adverse reactions or interactions

Diagnoses

- Ineffective protection
- Ineffective health maintenance
- Deficient knowledge

Planning Goals

- Patient shows signs of improvement
- No infections or complications arise
- Patient and family understand the drug regimen

Implementation

- Reconstitute and give IV as directed—use local anesthetic if needed for injection-site pain
- Discard solution if opaque or contains particles
- May be given intravesically (into the bladder): dehydrate patient first, then administer slowly over 2 hours once weekly for 4 weeks
- Can also be given intracavitarily
- Store powder in the fridge, away from sunlight
- Stop therapy if WBC < 3,000/μL or platelets < 150,000/μL
- Use allopurinol + hydration to prevent uric acid buildup
- Advise breastfeeding patients to stop during treatment

Evaluation

- Cancer shows improvement
- Patient remains free of infection and bleeding
- Patient and family show clear understanding of therapy

Alkylating-like Drugs: Platinum-Based Chemotherapy

These drugs contain platinum and act similarly to traditional alkylating agents by cross-linking DNA and stopping cancer cell growth. Common ones include:

- Carboplatin
- Cisplatin
- Oxaliplatin

Uses

- Carboplatin: ovarian and lung cancers
- Cisplatin: testicular, bladder, ovarian, head, neck, and lung cancers
- Oxaliplatin: used with other drugs to treat colorectal cancer

How They Work

These drugs are cell cycle–nonspecific and form DNA cross-links to prevent replication. They reach high concentrations in organs like the kidneys, liver, intestines, and testes, but don't cross into the brain easily.

Adverse Reactions

- Bone marrow suppression (carboplatin)
- Kidney toxicity (especially with cisplatin)
- Neurotoxicity, more so with cisplatin
- Hearing loss and tinnitus (mainly with cisplatin)
- Nausea and vomiting, which can be severe and prolonged

Drug Interactions

- Risk of kidney toxicity increases when taken with aminoglycosides
- Risk of hearing loss rises with diuretics like furosemide
- Cisplatin may lower phenytoin levels

Nursing Process

Assessment

- Evaluate CBC, electrolytes (especially potassium and magnesium), renal function, and audiometry results
- Watch for signs of toxicity or drug interactions
- Assess the patient's overall condition and response to treatment

Diagnoses

- Ineffective protection (from low blood counts)

397

- Risk for renal impairment or hearing loss
- Deficient knowledge

Planning Goals

- Patient improves based on testing
- No signs of infection, kidney damage, or hearing loss
- Patient and family understand therapy and precautions

Implementation

- Hydrate well before and after cisplatin
- Use chloride-containing solutions for cisplatin—avoid aluminum-containing IV equipment
- Monitor renal function closely—don't repeat dose if kidney markers are off
- Anti-nausea meds (ondansetron, granisetron, metoclopramide) can be used before and after therapy
- For delayed vomiting (3–5 days later), continue antiemetics
- Add potassium chloride to IV fluids to prevent hypokalemia
- Watch for anaphylaxis—have emergency drugs ready
- Teach patient to report tinnitus, swelling, or low urine output

Evaluation

- Cancer shows improvement
- No infections, kidney damage, or hearing loss
- Patient and caregiver fully understand therapy and monitoring needs

14.3. Antimetabolite drugs

Antimetabolite drugs are designed to mimic natural building blocks of DNA. Because they resemble the body's own DNA base pairs, they can sneak into the processes that build nucleic acids and proteins—essential components of all cells, including cancer cells.

Getting Specific

What makes antimetabolites especially effective is their targeted action. These drugs are S phase–specific, meaning they focus on cells that are actively copying DNA. Since cancer cells tend to divide quickly, they're especially vulnerable to these medications. However, normal cells that reproduce rapidly—like those in the bone marrow, GI tract, and hair follicles—can also be affected.

Types of Antimetabolites

Antimetabolites are grouped based on which natural metabolites they imitate:

- Folic acid analogues
- Pyrimidine analogues
- Purine analogues

Folic Acid Analogues: Methotrexate

Although many folic acid analogues have been developed, methotrexate remains the gold standard. It's one of the most widely used drugs in cancer therapy—and even in certain non-cancer conditions.

How It Works (Pharmacodynamics)

Methotrexate blocks the enzyme dihydrofolate reductase, which is essential for processing folic acid. Without folic acid, DNA and RNA synthesis grinds to a halt—leading to cell death.

How the Body Handles It (Pharmacokinetics)

- Absorbed well and distributed widely
- Tends to accumulate in body fluids like ascites or pleural effusion, which can prolong elimination and increase toxicity
- Partially metabolized in the liver but mostly excreted unchanged in urine
- Has a three-phase elimination pattern: rapid distribution, kidney clearance, and a terminal half-life (3–10 hours for low doses, 8–15 hours for high doses)

When It's Used (Pharmacotherapeutics)

Methotrexate is used to treat:

- Acute lymphoblastic and lymphocytic leukemia, especially in children
- Meningeal leukemia (given intrathecally)
- CNS tumors
- Choriocarcinoma
- Osteogenic sarcoma
- Lymphomas
- Cancers of the head, neck, bladder, testis, and breast

It's also used at lower doses for conditions like severe psoriasis, graft-versus-host disease, and rheumatoid arthritis when other treatments fail.

Drug Interactions to Watch

- Probenecid, NSAIDs, salicylates, and penicillin can increase methotrexate levels → higher risk of toxicity
- Alcohol increases the risk of liver damage
- Trimethoprim-sulfamethoxazole may cause serious blood cell abnormalities
- Cholestyramine can reduce absorption

Adverse Effects

- Bone marrow suppression
- Stomatitis (painful mouth inflammation)
- Pulmonary toxicity (pneumonitis or fibrosis)
- Photosensitivity and hair loss
- Kidney toxicity, especially at high doses

Leucovorin rescue (folinic acid) is often used with high-dose methotrexate to reduce harmful side effects.

Intrathecal administration can cause seizures, paralysis, and even death—less severe effects may include headache, fever, neck stiffness, and irritability.

Nursing Process: Methotrexate

Assessment

- Full baseline assessment and frequent reassessment
- Monitor I&O, vital signs, and IV site
- Check labs: CBC, liver and kidney function, uric acid
- Evaluate understanding of the drug plan

Diagnoses

- Ineffective protection (from side effects)
- Risk for infection (due to immune suppression)
- Knowledge deficit

Planning Goals

- Prevent serious complications
- Prevent infection
- Ensure patient and caregiver understand therapy

Implementation

- Follow safe handling protocols
- Offer antiemetics before treatment
- Provide regular oral care to prevent mouth sores
- Anticipate leucovorin use during high-dose therapy
- Educate patients to avoid immunizations until blood counts stabilize

Evaluation

- No serious complications occur
- No signs of infection
- Patient and family understand the drug regimen

Pyrimidine Analogues

These drugs disrupt the production of pyrimidine nucleotides, which are vital for making DNA. Examples include:

- Capecitabine
- Cytarabine
- Floxuridine
- Fluorouracil (5-FU)
- Gemcitabine

Pharmacokinetics

- Poor oral absorption, so usually given IV (except capecitabine)
- Distributed widely, often reaching CSF
- Metabolized in the liver, excreted in urine
- Intrathecal cytarabine is often used for CNS leukemia

Pharmacodynamics

They mimic pyrimidine structures and interfere with DNA synthesis, leading to cell death.

Pharmacotherapeutics

Used to treat:

- Acute leukemias
- GI tract cancers (colorectal, pancreatic, stomach, esophageal)
- Breast and ovarian cancer
- Lymphomas

Drug Interactions (Mainly with Capecitabine)

- Antacids may increase absorption
- May increase warfarin effects → bleeding risk
- Can raise phenytoin levels

Adverse Effects

- Fatigue
- Mucositis (mouth, throat, and GI tract irritation)
- Bone marrow suppression
- Nausea and anorexia
- Hand-foot syndrome, especially with high-dose cytarabine

High-dose cytarabine may cause neurotoxicity, chemical conjunctivitis, or diarrhea.

Fluorouracil often causes diarrhea and hair loss.

Nursing Process: Pyrimidine Analogues

Assessment

- Baseline assessment and ongoing monitoring
- Track fluid status, labs, and IV site
- Watch closely for toxicity—especially hand-foot syndrome

Diagnoses

- Ineffective protection
- Risk for infection
- Knowledge deficit

Planning Goals

- Minimize drug complications
- Prevent infection
- Ensure patient and family understand treatment

Implementation

- Safe handling and administration
- Antiemetics to manage nausea
- Use allopurinol with cytarabine to reduce uric acid buildup
- Promote oral hygiene and hydration

- Stop the drug and notify the prescriber if stomatitis or diarrhea develop

Evaluation

- Patient avoids serious toxicity
- No signs of infection
- Therapy is well understood

Purine Analogues

These agents mimic purine bases and interfere with both DNA and RNA production. They include:

- Cladribine
- Fludarabine phosphate
- Mercaptopurine
- Pentostatin
- Thioguanine

How They Work

After being converted to their active form inside the cell, these drugs:

- Disrupt nucleic acid synthesis
- Inhibit enzymes involved in cell division
- Are S phase–specific, like pyrimidine analogues

Pentostatin, for example, blocks adenosine deaminase, which is highly active in T-cell leukemias.

When They're Used

Purine analogues are used for:

- Acute and chronic leukemias
- Lymphomas, especially of the lymphoid lineage

Drug Interactions

- Fludarabine + pentostatin may cause fatal lung toxicity

- Pentostatin + allopurinol may increase rash risk
- Mercaptopurine + allopurinol increases the risk of bone marrow suppression

Adverse Effects

- Bone marrow suppression
- Nausea, vomiting, mild diarrhea, anorexia
- Stomatitis
- Elevated uric acid from cell breakdown
- High-dose fludarabine can lead to blindness, coma, or death

Nursing Process: Purine Analogues

Assessment

- Full baseline and regular reassessment
- Watch for neutropenia and thrombocytopenia
- Monitor I&O, labs, and IV site

Diagnoses

- Ineffective protection
- Risk of infection
- Deficient knowledge

Planning Goals

- Avoid complications from therapy
- Prevent infections
- Ensure full understanding by patient and caregivers

Implementation

- Use safe handling procedures; these drugs pose mutagenic and carcinogenic risks to staff
- Provide antiemetics for nausea
- Delay immunizations until blood counts are safe
- Treat extravasation immediately

- No serious bleeding or infection
- Patient understands the therapy and knows what to report

14.4. Antibiotic antineoplastic drugs

Antibiotic antineoplastic drugs are unique because they come from microbial sources but are used not to fight bacteria—but to destroy cancer cells. These medications work by binding to DNA, disrupting key processes in both cancerous and normal cells. Despite the name "antibiotic," their real target here is tumor destruction.

These powerful agents include:

- Anthracyclines: daunorubicin, doxorubicin, epirubicin, idarubicin
- Bleomycin
- Dactinomycin
- Mitomycin
- Mitoxantrone

How They're Given (Pharmacokinetics)

Most of these drugs are given intravenously (IV), which means they skip the digestive system and go directly into the bloodstream—making them 100% bioavailable.

Some can also be delivered directly into specific areas, like:

- Bladder installations (e.g., mitomycin, doxorubicin, bleomycin)
- Pleural space (e.g., bleomycin, for treating malignant effusions)

Bleomycin, when used in the pleural space, can be partially absorbed—up to 50% of the dose.

Distribution, metabolism, and elimination vary by drug and by individual, so monitoring is essential.

How They Work (Pharmacodynamics)

Most of these drugs intercalate into the DNA—this means they slip between the rungs of the DNA ladder (base pairs), physically forcing them apart. When the cell tries to copy its DNA, this interference causes errors—mutant DNA that can't support cell survival.

Mitomycin, on the other hand, behaves like an alkylating agent. Once inside the cell, it causes DNA cross-linking, strand breaks, and inhibits replication, all of which lead to cell death.

What They Treat (Pharmacotherapeutics)

These drugs are used in a wide range of cancers, including:

- Hodgkin's disease and other lymphomas
- Testicular carcinoma
- Squamous cell carcinoma (head, neck, cervix)
- Wilms' tumor (in children)
- Osteogenic sarcoma, rhabdomyosarcoma, Ewing's sarcoma
- Breast, ovarian, bladder, and lung cancer
- Melanoma and GI tract cancers
- Choriocarcinoma, acute leukemia, neuroblastoma

Drug Interactions

Because these drugs are often used in combination therapies, interactions are important to monitor:

- Fludarabine + idarubicin: Not recommended—can cause fatal lung toxicity
- Bleomycin may lower digoxin and phenytoin levels
- Doxorubicin may also reduce digoxin levels
- Combination therapy may increase leukopenia and thrombocytopenia
- Mitomycin + vinca alkaloids: Risk of acute respiratory distress
- Herbal products like St. John's wort and black cohosh may lower doxorubicin levels

Adverse Reactions

The most common side effects include:

- Bone marrow suppression (lowered blood counts)
- Irreversible heart damage (cardiomyopathy), especially with anthracyclines
- Nausea and vomiting

Special precautions with bleomycin:

- Pre-medicate with antihistamines and antipyretics to prevent fever and chills
- Give test doses in lymphoma patients to reduce the risk of anaphylaxis

Color changes:

- Doxorubicin, daunorubicin, epirubicin, and idarubicin may turn urine red
- Mitoxantrone can cause blue-green urine

Nursing Process: Antibiotic Antineoplastics

Assessment

- Full assessment before therapy begins
- Review patient history and cancer type
- Monitor ECG before using doxorubicin or daunorubicin
- Track labs: CBC, platelets, liver enzymes (ALT, AST), bilirubin, kidney markers (BUN, creatinine, uric acid), and hemoglobin
- Monitor lung function regularly in patients on bleomycin
- Ensure IV or catheter sites remain patent and irritation-free

Key Nursing Diagnoses

- Ineffective health maintenance related to cancer
- Risk for infection due to low WBCs
- Deficient knowledge about the treatment plan

Planning Outcome Goals

- Patient shows improvement in their condition
- No signs of infection (normal temperature, WBC count, negative cultures)
- Patient and caregivers understand the drug regimen and precautions

Implementation

- Follow all safety protocols for chemotherapy preparation and disposal
- Provide emotional support to reduce patient and family anxiety
- Keep epinephrine, corticosteroids, and antihistamines on hand in case of anaphylaxis
- Treat extravasation immediately
- Ensure adequate hydration, especially during idarubicin therapy

Evaluation

- Patient shows measurable improvement in response to treatment
- No infections or treatment-related complications occur
- Patient and family demonstrate understanding of how the medication works and what to report

14.5. Hormonal Antineoplastic Drugs and Hormone Modulators

Hormonal therapies and hormone modulators are used to slow down or block the growth of certain cancers—or to manage their symptoms—by interfering with the body's hormone signals. These drugs either mimic or block hormones to stop tumor growth, especially in cancers that are hormone-sensitive.

They're grouped into six major classes:

- Aromatase inhibitors
- Antiestrogens

- Androgens
- Antiandrogens
- Progestins
- Gonadotropin-releasing hormone (GnRH) analogues

Targeting Hormone-Dependent Cancers

Hormonal drugs are especially effective against cancers that rely on hormones to grow—like breast, prostate, and endometrial cancers. Corticosteroids are also used in some leukemias and lymphomas because of their effects on immune cells like lymphocytes.

Aromatase Inhibitors

These drugs stop androgens (male hormones) from being converted into estrogen in postmenopausal women. Since many breast cancers are fueled by estrogen, blocking this pathway helps prevent cancer cells from multiplying.

Examples:

- Type 1 (steroidal): Exemestane
- Type 2 (nonsteroidal): Anastrozole, Letrozole

How They Work

After menopause, estrogen is mainly produced in fat and muscle tissues via the aromatase enzyme. Aromatase inhibitors lower estrogen levels, cutting off the fuel supply to estrogen-sensitive tumors. However, long-term use can reduce bone density and lead to osteoporosis.

- Type 1 inhibitors bind irreversibly to the aromatase enzyme
- Type 2 inhibitors bind reversibly

How They're Used

Prescribed primarily for postmenopausal women with metastatic breast cancer, either alone or alongside drugs like tamoxifen.

Watch Out For

- Tamoxifen and estrogen-containing products can reduce effectiveness
- CYP3A4 inducers (like certain anticonvulsants or antibiotics) can lower exemestane levels

Side Effects

Most are mild: dizziness, hot flashes, joint pain, fatigue, mild nausea, and urinary infections. They may also raise cholesterol levels.

Nursing Process – Aromatase Inhibitors

Assessment

- Assess cancer status and monitor for side effects
- Watch for GI issues and hydration status

Diagnoses

- Ineffective health maintenance
- Risk of adverse effects
- Deficient knowledge

Planning & Implementation

- Educate patient and family
- Avoid giving with estrogen products
- Administer after meals

Evaluation

- Positive treatment response
- No serious side effects
- Family understands therapy plan

Antiestrogens

These drugs block estrogen receptors, stopping estrogen from stimulating cancer growth.

Examples:

- Tamoxifen, Toremifene (agonist-antagonists)
- Fulvestrant (pure antagonist)

How They Work

They bind to estrogen receptors on cancer cells, preventing estrogen from stimulating DNA synthesis and cell growth—especially in breast cancer. Tamoxifen also acts as an estrogen agonist in bones, which helps maintain bone density.

Uses

- Tamoxifen: Adjuvant and palliative therapy for estrogen receptor–positive breast cancer, including prevention in high-risk women
- Toremifene: Used in metastatic breast cancer
- Fulvestrant: For advanced cases that no longer respond to tamoxifen

Drug Interactions

- Tamoxifen and toremifene may increase the effect of warfarin
- Bromocriptine increases tamoxifen's effects
- Fulvestrant has no major interactions

Side Effects

- Tamoxifen: Hot flashes, GI issues, fluid retention, blood count changes, and hypercalcemia if bone metastasis is present
- Toremifene: Similar to tamoxifen with more vaginal symptoms
- Fulvestrant: GI discomfort, headache, back pain, pharyngitis

Nursing Process – Antiestrogens

Assessment

- Monitor CBC, lipids, and calcium levels
- Assess for drug side effects and hydration

Diagnoses

- Health maintenance challenges
- Risk for dehydration
- Deficient knowledge

Planning & Implementation

- Swallow tablets whole (don't crush)
- Watch for bleeding with warfarin use
- Teach about ongoing monitoring

Evaluation

- Patient maintains hydration
- Cancer symptoms improve
- Patient understands treatment

Androgens

Synthetic male hormones used to slow the growth of breast cancer in postmenopausal women, especially when cancer has spread to the bones.

Examples:

- Fluoxymesterone, Testolactone, Testosterone enanthate, Testosterone propionate

How They Work

They reduce the number of estrogen receptors or compete with estrogen at the receptor site, helping block estrogen-driven tumor growth.

How They're Used

Given orally or intramuscularly, often weekly. IM injections are designed for slow absorption and longer duration of action.

Drug Interactions

May alter insulin, anticoagulant, or oral antidiabetic drug effects. Combined with other liver-toxic drugs, they raise the risk of liver toxicity.

Side Effects

- Common: Nausea, vomiting, fluid retention, tingling
- In women: Acne, deeper voice, breast and clitoral enlargement, menstrual changes, increased body hair

Nursing Process – Androgens

Assessment

- Monitor breast cancer status, labs (especially calcium), and side effects

Diagnoses

- Ineffective health maintenance
- Sensory disturbances
- Knowledge deficit

Planning & Implementation

- Encourage fluid intake and physical activity
- Note: It may take up to 3 months to notice results

Evaluation

- Patient feels better
- Patient understands safety precautions for side effects

Antiandrogens

Used in prostate cancer, these drugs block the effects of male hormones (androgens) on tumor cells.

Examples:

- Flutamide, Nilutamide, Bicalutamide

How They Work

They prevent testosterone from binding to receptors in the prostate, helping shrink the tumor.

How They're Used

Used with a gonadotropin-releasing hormone analogue (like leuprolide) to reduce testosterone production and block its action—a dual approach to starving the tumor.

Drug Interactions

Minimal. May slightly increase bleeding risk with warfarin.

Side Effects

- Hot flashes
- Loss of libido
- Impotence
- Breast enlargement
- Unusual urine colors (e.g., blue-green with flutamide)

Nursing Process – Antiandrogens

Assessment

- Monitor prostate cancer progression, liver function, hydration

Diagnoses

- Health maintenance challenges
- Fluid volume risk
- Knowledge deficit

Planning & Implementation

- Take the meds consistently—don't stop flutamide or leuprolide
- Teach injection techniques if patient is self-administering

Evaluation

- Patient shows improvement

- Maintains hydration
- Understands dual-drug regimen

Progestins

These hormones are used palliatively to manage breast, renal, and endometrial cancers.

Examples:

- Megestrol acetate, Medroxyprogesterone acetate

How They Work

The exact mechanism isn't fully understood, but progestins likely bind to hormone receptors, slowing the growth of hormone-sensitive tumors.

They are cytostatic, meaning they stop cells from multiplying, rather than killing them outright.

Side Effects

- Fluid retention
- Thromboembolism
- Menstrual changes
- Acne, breast tenderness
- Liver function abnormalities

Some may have allergic reactions to the injection oil (e.g., sesame or castor oil).

Nursing Process – Progestins

Assessment

- Check injection sites, labs, and for allergic reactions

Diagnoses

- Fluid imbalance
- Health maintenance issues

- Knowledge deficit

Planning & Implementation

- Rotate injection sites
- Avoid smoking and caffeine
- Teach breast self-exams

Evaluation

- No fluid imbalances
- Cancer symptoms improve
- Patient understands therapy

Gonadotropin-Releasing Hormone (GnRH) Analogues

Used in advanced prostate cancer to suppress testosterone production without surgery.

Examples:

- Goserelin, Leuprolide, Triptorelin

How They Work

Initially, these drugs cause a temporary surge in testosterone (called a "flare"), followed by suppression of testosterone levels to levels similar to surgical castration. This reduces hormone-driven tumor growth.

Side Effects

- Hot flashes
- Loss of libido
- GI upset
- Temporary worsening of symptoms during the first 2 weeks
- Bone pain may increase temporarily

Nursing Process – GnRH Analogues

Assessment

- Monitor for pain flare or worsening symptoms at the start of therapy

Diagnoses

- Acute pain
- Knowledge deficit
- Ineffective health maintenance

Planning & Implementation

- Administer as prescribed (injection or implant)
- Avoid aspiration with injection
- Schedule timely follow-ups (e.g., every 28 days for implants)
- Teach subcut techniques for home administration

Evaluation

- Patient reports improvement
- Pain is managed
- Family understands treatment and reporting schedule

14.6. Natural Antineoplastic Drugs

Natural antineoplastic drugs are derived from plant sources and are used to target and destroy cancer cells. Two key groups in this category include:

- Vinca alkaloids
- Podophyllotoxins

Vinca Alkaloids

These drugs come from the periwinkle plant and specifically target the M phase of the cell cycle, the stage where cells divide. Examples include:

- Vinblastine

- Vincristine
- Vinorelbine

How They Move Through the Body (Pharmacokinetics)

Given IV, these drugs spread throughout the body, are partially metabolized in the liver, and are mostly eliminated through the feces. Only a small amount is excreted in urine.

How They Work (Pharmacodynamics)

Vinca alkaloids interfere with microtubules, which are like the scaffolding inside cells that help organize DNA during division. They bind to tubulin, a key structural protein.

When the microtubules can't function properly, chromosomes can't align or separate, so cell division gets stuck in metaphase, leading to cell death. These drugs are M phase–specific and can also affect cell movement, immune responses, and even nerve function.

What They're Used For (Pharmacotherapeutics)

- Vinblastine: Testicular cancer, lymphomas, Kaposi's sarcoma, neuroblastoma, breast cancer, choriocarcinoma
- Vincristine: Leukemias, Hodgkin's and non-Hodgkin's lymphomas, Wilms' tumor, rhabdomyosarcoma
- Vinorelbine: Non–small-cell lung cancer, metastatic breast cancer, cisplatin-resistant ovarian cancer, Hodgkin's disease

Drug Interactions

- Erythromycin can increase vinblastine's toxicity
- Phenytoin levels may drop when taken with vinblastine
- Vincristine reduces the effect of digoxin
- Asparaginase raises vincristine toxicity
- Calcium channel blockers may increase vincristine accumulation and its side effects

Side Effects

- Nausea, vomiting, constipation, and stomatitis
- Bone marrow suppression (especially with vinblastine and vinorelbine)
- Nerve problems—like tingling, numbness, and weakness—are common with vincristine
- Tumor pain (especially with vinblastine), described as stinging or burning
- Hair loss (reversible, and more likely with vincristine)

Nursing Process – Vinca Alkaloids

Assessment

- Evaluate the patient's condition regularly
- Watch for acute bronchospasm, especially if also receiving mitomycin
- Assess for numbness, tingling, gait changes, footdrop, or wristdrop
- Monitor for constipation—an early sign of neurotoxicity
- Keep an eye on uric acid levels, especially in leukemia or lymphoma patients

Diagnoses

- Ineffective health maintenance
- Risk for injury (neurotoxicity, leukopenia)
- Deficient knowledge of therapy

Planning & Implementation

- Administer antiemetics before dosing
- Prepare and handle according to safety guidelines—these are hazardous drugs
- Stop infusion immediately if extravasation or bronchospasm occurs
- Maintain adequate fluid intake to help flush out uric acid

- Delay next dose if bilirubin >3 mg/dL or hold for a week to prevent severe leukopenia

Evaluation

- Patient shows clinical improvement
- No serious hematologic complications
- Patient and family understand treatment and precautions

Podophyllotoxins

These are semisynthetic glycosides that work during the G2 and late S phases of the cell cycle. They include:

- Etoposide
- Teniposide

How They Move (Pharmacokinetics)

- Moderately absorbed orally
- Widely distributed but don't reach the CSF well
- Metabolized in the liver and excreted mostly through urine

How They Work (Pharmacodynamics)

Though not fully understood, podophyllotoxins work by:

- Blocking cells in late S or G2 phase (depending on concentration)
- Causing single-strand breaks in DNA
- Inhibiting nucleotide transport and DNA building blocks

What They're Used For (Pharmacotherapeutics)

- Etoposide: Testicular cancer, small-cell lung cancer
- Teniposide: Childhood leukemia that doesn't respond to other treatments

Drug Interactions

- Teniposide may affect methotrexate levels

- Etoposide increases bleeding risk with warfarin
- St. John's wort lowers both drug levels

Side Effects

- Hair loss (common but reversible)
- Nausea, vomiting, anorexia, stomatitis
- Bone marrow suppression (watch for leukopenia)
- Low blood pressure during rapid IV infusion—infuse slowly!

Nursing Process – Podophyllotoxins

Assessment

- Baseline and regular assessment during therapy
- Monitor blood pressure every 30 minutes during infusion
- Track tumor size, response to therapy, and lab values (especially CBC)
- Watch for signs of infection and bleeding

Diagnoses

- Ineffective health maintenance
- Risk for hematologic complications
- Deficient knowledge

Planning & Implementation

- Store oral capsules in the fridge
- Infuse over at least 30 minutes to avoid hypotension
- Don't use in-line membrane filters (the diluent dissolves them!)
- Keep emergency meds (diphenhydramine, epinephrine, hydrocortisone) on hand
- Teach patient about hair loss, infection precautions, and when to report symptoms
- Stop the infusion if systolic BP drops below 90 mm Hg

Evaluation

- Patient tolerates treatment well

- No serious complications from blood count suppression
- Patient and family can explain the purpose of therapy and precautions

14.7. Monoclonal antibodies

Thanks to breakthroughs in recombinant DNA technology, we now have monoclonal antibodies—lab-created molecules designed to target specific proteins on cancer or immune cells. These precision therapies help the body's immune system recognize and attack cancer cells more effectively.

Examples include:

- Ibritumomab tiuxetan
- Nivolumab
- Dinutuximab
- Rituximab
- Trastuzumab

How They Move (Pharmacokinetics)

Monoclonal antibodies are large protein molecules, so they can't be absorbed orally—they must be given by injection. Once in the body, they typically stay in the bloodstream or targeted tissues and can have long half-lives, sometimes lasting weeks.

How They Work (Pharmacodynamics)

These antibodies are designed to lock onto specific targets—either receptors on cancer cells or proteins involved in tumor growth. Once attached, they can:

- Trigger cell death (apoptosis)
- Flag cancer cells for immune attack
- Disrupt tumor growth pathways

Some, like ibritumomab tiuxetan, even carry radioactive particles directly to the tumor, delivering a localized radiation dose.

When They're Used (Pharmacotherapeutics)

Monoclonal antibodies are powerful tools for treating both solid tumors and blood cancers:

- Rituximab and ibritumomab tiuxetan target CD20 on B-cell lymphomas (like non-Hodgkin's)
- Trastuzumab zeroes in on HER2 receptors in breast cancer
- Nivolumab targets PD-1 in melanoma
- Dinutuximab binds GD2 in pediatric neuroblastoma

Drug Interactions

Nivolumab and dinutuximab: No known interactions

Ibritumomab: May increase risk of bleeding and interact with warfarin, NSAIDs, clopidogrel, and immunosuppressants

Trastuzumab: Can worsen heart toxicity if given with anthracyclines

Rituximab: When combined with cisplatin, may increase kidney damage

Adverse Reactions

The most common side effects are infusion-related, and may include:

- Fever and chills
- Low blood pressure
- Shortness of breath
- Anaphylaxis (in rare cases, fatal)

Some agents have specific risks:

- Ibritumomab tiuxetan can cause myelosuppression, increasing infection risk
- Rituximab + cisplatin increases the risk of renal toxicity
- Trastuzumab increases risk of cardiac complications

Nursing Process – Monoclonal Antibodies

Assessment

- Evaluate patient's condition and treatment goals regularly

- Monitor vital signs before and during infusions—watch for hypotension
- Track tumor size, growth rate, and response through labs and imaging
- Check CBC and platelet count before starting and weekly during therapy
- Monitor for hematologic toxicity, such as myelosuppression
- Assess renal function (especially with rituximab + cisplatin)
- Monitor CD4+ count post-treatment until it's over 200 cells/μL
- Check liver function during dinutuximab therapy
- Ensure patient and family understand the treatment plan

Diagnoses

- Risk for infection due to immunosuppression
- Fatigue related to treatment
- Deficient knowledge about drug therapy

Planning Goals

- No signs of infection (normal WBCs, temp, and cultures)
- Fatigue is minimized and manageable
- Patient and family demonstrate understanding of the drug regimen

Implementation Tips

- Reconstitute and administer according to facility protocol
- Discard solutions if discolored or containing particles
- Use a 5-micron filter when preparing
- Irradiate blood if transfusion is needed (to prevent graft-versus-host disease)
- Avoid live vaccines during treatment
- If therapy is paused for more than 7 days, restart at a lower dose

- Rituximab and trastuzumab must be given slow IV infusion (not bolus or IV push)
- Infuse over at least 2 hours to reduce risk of adverse reactions
- Teach patients to use effective contraception during and for 6 months after therapy

Evaluation

- Patient remains free from infection
- Patient can perform daily activities
- Patient and family can explain medication purpose, side effects, and safety measures

14.8. Topoisomerase I inhibitors

As the name implies, topoisomerase I inhibitors inhibit the enzyme topoisomerase I. These agents are derived from a naturally occurring alkaloid from the Chinese tree Camptotheca acuminata. Currently available drugs include:

- irinotecan
- topotecan.

Pharmacokinetics

Irinotecan and topotecan are minimally absorbed and must be given IV. Irinotecan undergoes metabolic changes to become the active metabolite SN-38. The half-life of SN-38 is approximately 10 hours, and it's eliminated through biliary excretion.

Topotecan is metabolized hepatically, although renal excretion is a significant elimination pathway.

Pharmacodynamics

These agents exert their cytotoxic effect by inhibiting the topoisomerase I enzyme, an essential enzyme that mediates the relaxation of supercoiled DNA. Topoisomerase inhibitors bind to the DNA topoisomerase I complex and prevent resealing, thereby causing DNA strand breaks, resulting in impaired DNA synthesis.

Pharmacotherapeutics

Topoisomerase I inhibitors are active against solid tumors and hematologic malignancies. Topotecan is administered for ovarian cancer, small-cell lung cancer, and acute myeloid leukemia. Irinotecan is administered to patients with colorectal cancer or small-cell lung cancer.

Drug interactions

Irinotecan is associated with the following drug interactions:

- Ketoconazole can significantly increase SN-38 serum concentrations when given with irinotecan, increasing the risk of associated toxicities.
- Concurrent administration of diuretics may exacerbate dehydration caused by irinotecan-induced diarrhea.
- Concurrent administration of laxatives with irinotecan can induce diarrhea.
- Prochlorperazine administered with irinotecan can increase the incidence of extrapyramidal toxicities.

Adverse reactions

Diarrhea is the most common adverse reaction to topoisomerase I inhibitors, especially irinotecan, which is cholinergically mediated; this can be reversed with atropine.

Delayed reaction

Late-onset diarrhea, which may persist for up to 1 week, can occur several days after chemotherapy has been administered. Treatment consists of loperamide given every 2 hours until stools become formed.

Common conditions, part two

Besides diarrhea, the more common adverse reactions to topoisomerase I inhibitors, particularly irinotecan, include:

- increased sweating and saliva production
- watery eyes
- abdominal cramps

- nausea and vomiting
- loss of appetite
- fatigue
- hair loss or thinning.

Only occasional

Occasionally, these reactions may occur:

- mouth sores and ulcers
- muscle cramps
- temporary effect on liver function tests
- rashes, which may be itchy.

Serious situation

These reactions rarely occur but are more serious:

- Both drugs are associated with significant myelosuppression, especially topotecan.
- Irinotecan has been associated with thromboembolic events, namely, myocardial infarction and stroke, which have resulted in death.

Nursing process

These nursing process steps are appropriate for patients undergoing treatment with topoisomerase I inhibitors.

Assessment

- Assess the patient's condition before therapy and regularly thereafter.
- Monitor the patient for adverse reactions and drug interactions.
- Obtain a baseline neutrophil count; it must be greater than 1,500 cells/µL and the patient's platelet count greater than 100,000 cells/µL before therapy can start.
- Frequent monitoring of the peripheral blood cell count is critical. Don't give repeated doses until the neutrophil count is greater than 1,000 cells/µL, platelet count is greater than

100,000 cells/μL, and hemoglobin level is greater than 9 mg/dL.

- Evaluate the patient's and family's knowledge of drug therapy.

Key nursing diagnoses

- Ineffective health maintenance related to the presence of neoplastic disease
- Ineffective protection related to drug-induced adverse reactions
- Deficient knowledge related to drug therapy

Planning outcome goals

- The patient will demonstrate an improvement in assessment findings and diagnostic testing.
- The risk of injury to the patient will be minimized.
- The patient and family will demonstrate an understanding of drug therapy.

Implementation

- Prepare the drug under a vertical laminar flow hood while wearing gloves and protective clothing. If the drug contacts skin, wash immediately and thoroughly with soap and water. If mucous membranes are affected, flush with water.
- Reconstitute the drug as ordered. Dilute and administer the drug according to facility policy.
- Give a topotecan IV infusion slowly, over at least 30 minutes; give an irinotecan IV infusion over at least 90 minutes.
- Protect unopened vials of the drug from light.
- Monitor the patient for signs and symptoms of infection, such as sore throat, fever, chills, or unusual bleeding or bruising, and report them promptly.
- Teach a female patient of childbearing age to avoid pregnancy and breast-feeding during treatment.

- Patient responds well to drug therapy.
- Patient doesn't develop serious complications from adverse hematologic reactions.
- Patient and family state an understanding of drug therapy.

14.9. Targeted therapies

A groundbreaking approach to anticancer therapies is to target proteins associated with the growth patterns for a specific type of cancer. These targeted therapies include epidermal growth factor receptor inhibitors (cetuximab, panitumumab, lenvatinib, and erlotinib), tyrosine inhibitors (gefitinib, imatinib, dasatinib, and nilotinib), vascular endothelial growth factor inhibitors (sunitinib and sorafenib), and the protease inhibitor bortezomib.

Pharmacokinetics

Gefitinib is available in an oral form of which approximately half the dose is absorbed. The drug is widely distributed in tissues. It undergoes hepatic metabolism with minimal urinary excretion.

Imatinib is available in an oral form, which is almost completely absorbed. It's 95% bound to plasma proteins and extensively metabolized by the liver. The half-life is approximately 15 hours.

Bortezomib isn't absorbed orally and must be given IV. It is extensively distributed into body tissues and hepatically metabolized.

Pharmacodynamics

Gefitinib inhibits the epidermal growth factor receptor-1 tyrosine kinase, which is overexpressed with certain cancers, such as non–small-cell lung cancer. This blocks signaling pathways for the growth, survival, and metastasis of cancer.

In a bind

Imatinib binds to the adenosine triphosphate binding domain of the BCR-ABL protein, which stimulates other tyrosine kinase proteins to result in abnormally high production of WBCs in chronic myeloid leukemia. This binding of imatinib effectively shuts down the abnormal WBC production.

Feeling a bit inhibited . . .

Bortezomib inhibits proteasomes, which are integral to cell cycle function and promote tumor growth. Proteolysis by bortezomib results in the disruption of normal homeostatic mechanisms and leads to cell death.

Pharmacotherapeutics

Gefitinib is used as a single agent for patients with non–small-cell lung cancer that has failed to respond to two previous standard chemotherapy regimens. Imatinib is used to treat chronic myeloid leukemia, acute lymphoid leukemia, and GI stromal tumors. Bortezomib is used to treat multiple myeloma that has relapsed after standard chemotherapy. Lenvatinib is used to treat metastatic or locally advanced thyroid malignancy.

Drug interactions

Bortezomib, gefitinib, and imatinib have been associated with some drug interactions:

- Bortezomib, when taken with drugs that are inhibitors or inducers of CYP3A4, may cause either toxicities or reduced efficacy of these drugs. Inhibitors of CYP3A4 include amiodarone, cimetidine, erythromycin, diltiazem, disulfiram, fluoxetine, grapefruit juice, verapamil, zafirlukast, and zileuton. Inducers of CYP3A4 include amiodarone, carbamazepine, nevirapine, phenobarbital, phenytoin, and rifampin.
- Bortezomib, when taken with oral antidiabetic agents, may cause hypoglycemia or hyperglycemia in patients with diabetes.
- Plasma levels of gefitinib and imatinib are reduced, sometimes substantially, when these drugs are given with

carbamazepine, dexamethasone, phenobarbital, phenytoin, rifampin, or St. John's wort.

- Taking high doses of ranitidine with sodium bicarbonate together with gefitinib reduces gefitinib levels.
- Administration of gefitinib or imatinib with warfarin causes elevations in the international normalized ratio, increasing the risk of bleeding.
- Drugs that inhibit the CYP3A4 family (such as clarithromycin, erythromycin, itraconazole, and ketoconazole) when taken with imatinib may increase imatinib plasma levels.
- Imatinib administered with CYP3A4 inducers (carbamazepine, dexamethasone, phenobarbital, phenytoin, and rifampin) may increase the metabolism of imatinib and decrease imatinib levels.
- Imatinib given with simvastatin increases simvastatin levels about threefold.
- Imatinib increases plasma levels of other CYP3A4-metabolized drugs, such as triazolobenzodiazepines, dihydropyridine, calcium channel blockers, and certain HMG-CoA reductase inhibitors.

Adverse reactions

Toxicities have occurred from administration of targeted therapies. Women should avoid becoming pregnant during administration of these agents because animal studies have shown that they cross the placental barrier and have resulted in fetal harm and death.

Gefitinib

Adverse reactions to gefitinib include:

- skin rash
- diarrhea
- abnormal eyelash growth
- lung and liver damage.

Lenvatinib

Adverse reactions to lenvatinib include:

- hypertension
- abdominal pain, nausea, vomiting, diarrhea, stomatitis
- arthralgia.

Imatinib

Adverse reactions to imatinib include:

- edema (periorbital and lower limb), which may result in pulmonary edema, effusions, and heart or renal failure; management includes treatment with diuretics and supportive measures such as decreasing the dosage
- nausea, vomiting, liver function abnormalities, and myelosuppression (especially neutropenia and thrombocytopenia).

Bortezomib

The most common adverse reactions to bortezomib include asthenic conditions (fatigue, malaise, and weakness), nausea, diarrhea, appetite loss (anorexia), constipation, pyrexia, and vomiting.

Other reactions include:

- peripheral neuropathy, headache, low blood pressure, liver toxicity, thrombocytopenia, and renal toxicity
- cardiac toxicity (arrhythmias, such as bradycardia, ventricular tachycardia, atrial fibrillation, and atrial flutter; heart failure; myocardial ischemia and infarction; pulmonary edema; and pericardial effusion).

Depending on the severity of the reactions, the dosage may need to be reduced or the drug withheld until toxicity resolves. Severe reactions may require discontinuing the medication.

Nursing process

These nursing process steps are appropriate for patients undergoing treatment with targeted therapies.

Assessment

- Assess the patient's condition before therapy and regularly thereafter.
- Monitor the patient for adverse reactions and drug interactions.

Weighty issues

- Obtain a baseline weight before therapy and weigh the patient daily throughout therapy. Evaluate and treat unexpected and rapid weight gain.
- Evaluate the patient's and family's knowledge of drug therapy.

Key nursing diagnoses

- Ineffective health maintenance related to the presence of neoplastic disease
- Risk for falls related to drug-induced adverse reactions
- Deficient knowledge related to drug therapy

Planning outcome goals

- The patient will demonstrate an improvement in assessment findings and diagnostic testing.
- The risk of injury to the patient will be minimized.
- The patient and family will demonstrate an understanding of drug therapy.

Implementation

- Reconstitute the drug as ordered and administer according to facility policy.
- Monitor the patient closely for fluid retention, which can be severe.
- Monitor the patient's CBC weekly for the first month, biweekly for the second month, and periodically thereafter.
- Because GI irritation is common, give the drug with food as appropriate.

- Monitor liver function tests carefully because hepatotoxicity (occasionally severe) may occur. Decrease the dosage as needed.
- Because the long-term safety of the drug isn't known, monitor renal and liver function and immunosuppression carefully.

Evaluation

- Patient responds well to drug therapy.
- Patient doesn't develop serious complications from adverse reactions.
- Patient and family state an understanding of drug therapy.

14.10.   Unclassified antineoplastic drugs

Not all cancer-fighting medications fit neatly into one category. Some drugs work in unique ways or come from different backgrounds, and we group them together as "unclassified" antineoplastics. These include:

- Aldesleukin
- Asparaginases
- Hydroxyurea
- Interferons
- Procarbazine
- Taxanes (paclitaxel, docetaxel)

Aldesleukin

Aldesleukin is a man-made version of interleukin-2 (IL-2), a substance our immune system naturally produces. It's used mainly to treat metastatic renal cell carcinoma, and occasionally Kaposi's sarcoma or metastatic melanoma.

How It Works

Although we don't fully understand its antitumor action, aldesleukin seems to stimulate the immune system to attack cancer cells.

What to Expect

- Given through IV
- Quickly taken up by organs like the liver, kidneys, and lungs
- Most of it is cleared through the kidneys

Interactions to Watch

Aldesleukin can interact with:

- Sedatives, opioids, and tranquilizers (increasing drowsiness)
- Steroids (which may reduce its effectiveness)
- Blood pressure medications (amplifying hypotension)
- Other drugs toxic to the liver, kidneys, heart, or bone marrow

Possible Side Effects

- Pulmonary congestion, trouble breathing
- Changes in blood counts (anemia, low WBCs or platelets)
- Kidney issues, such as low urine output or high creatinine
- Liver enzyme elevation
- GI discomfort: nausea, vomiting, stomatitis
- Low calcium and magnesium levels
- Hypertension

Nursing Considerations

- Monitor blood counts and kidney function
- Watch for organ-specific toxicities
- Educate patient and caregivers on what to expect

Asparaginases (including pegaspargase)

These drugs exploit a difference between healthy and cancer cells. While normal cells make their own asparagine, some leukemia cells can't—and asparaginases starve those cancer cells of it.

How It Works

By breaking down asparagine, these drugs disrupt protein synthesis in cancer cells, ultimately killing them.

Uses

Primarily used for acute lymphocytic leukemia (ALL), often alongside other chemotherapy agents.

Interactions

- Reduces effectiveness of methotrexate
- Higher risk of side effects when used with prednisone or vincristine

Side Effects

- Allergic reactions and anaphylaxis (especially with intermittent IV dosing)
- Pancreatitis, coagulopathy, liver issues
- Nausea, vomiting, fever, headache
- Bone marrow suppression

Nursing Tips

- Have emergency supplies ready for anaphylaxis
- Monitor pancreatic enzymes (amylase/lipase)
- Give IV slowly (at least 30 minutes)
- Provide hydration and consider allopurinol to prevent uric acid build-up

Hydroxyurea

Hydroxyurea is a cell-cycle–specific drug commonly used for chronic myelogenous leukemia and occasionally for solid tumors like head and neck cancer.

How It Works

It blocks the enzyme ribonucleotide reductase, which cancer cells need to make DNA, leading to cell cycle arrest and death, especially in the S phase.

Absorption & Elimination

- Taken orally and well absorbed
- Metabolized in the liver and lungs
- Excreted via the kidneys

Interactions

- More toxic when combined with radiation or cytotoxic drugs

Side Effects

- Bone marrow suppression
- Liver toxicity
- Nausea, vomiting, drowsiness
- Elevated uric acid (may need allopurinol)

Nursing Tips

- Monitor blood counts and kidney function
- Encourage fluids to prevent kidney issues
- Educate on signs of infection and when to seek help
- Warn patients not to become pregnant during therapy

Interferons

These natural proteins—especially alpha interferons—are used to treat viral infections and some cancers like hairy cell leukemia and Kaposi's sarcoma.

How They Work

They don't kill cancer cells directly. Instead, they:

- Boost the immune response

- Inhibit viral replication
- Suppress tumor cell proliferation

Interactions

- May amplify effects of CNS depressants
- Interact with live vaccines
- Can increase risk of bone marrow suppression if used with other myelosuppressive treatments

Side Effects

- Flu-like symptoms (fatigue, chills, fever, muscle aches)
- GI upset
- Blood abnormalities (low WBCs, anemia)
- Heart and lung issues (hypotension, edema, heart failure)

Nursing Tips

- Premedicate with acetaminophen to ease flu-like symptoms
- Give at bedtime to reduce daytime fatigue
- Monitor CBC and hydration
- Store the drug properly (usually refrigerated)

Procarbazine

Used for Hodgkin's disease, lymphomas, and some brain tumors, procarbazine is a bit of an outlier: it works like an MAO inhibitor.

How It Works

After being activated in the liver, it interferes with DNA, RNA, and protein synthesis, which hampers cancer cell growth.

Interactions

- Dangerous with meperidine (can cause fatal hypotension)
- Interacts with tyramine-rich foods and CNS depressants
- Avoid alcohol and caffeine during treatment

Side Effects

- Bone marrow suppression
- Pulmonary fibrosis, interstitial pneumonitis
- Nausea, vomiting, stomatitis
- Flu-like symptoms

Nursing Tips

- Give at bedtime to reduce nausea
- Monitor for signs of CNS toxicity
- Educate patients to avoid certain foods and drugs
- Stop the drug and alert the provider if serious side effects occur

Taxanes (Paclitaxel and Docetaxel)

These plant-derived drugs are used for metastatic breast and ovarian cancers, and sometimes for head, neck, or lung cancers.

How They Work

Taxanes interfere with the microtubule structures inside cells, preventing them from dividing properly.

Interactions

- Metabolized by the liver; many drugs can affect their levels
- Cisplatin may increase side effects when used with paclitaxel

Side Effects

- Bone marrow suppression
- Allergic reactions
- Peripheral neuropathy, joint pain
- Nausea, vomiting, hair loss
- Fluid retention (more common with docetaxel)

Nursing Tips

- Premedicate with steroids and antihistamines

- Handle with care (these drugs are hazardous to staff too)
- Monitor for neuropathy, infection, and bleeding
- Remind patients that hair loss is common but reversible

Panobinostat

Panobinostat is a newer oral drug used in relapsed multiple myeloma, often combined with bortezomib and dexamethasone.

How It Works

It inhibits histone deacetylase, leading to cell cycle arrest and potentially cell death.

- **Side Effects**
- Fatigue
- Anemia
- Risk of QT prolongation (so monitor heart function carefully)

Palbociclib

This oral drug targets metastatic breast cancer in postmenopausal women with HER2-negative, hormone receptor-positive tumors. It's often paired with letrozole.

How It Works

Palbociclib blocks the enzymes CDK 4 and 6, halting cancer cell growth at a key phase of the cell cycle.

Interactions

- Affected by CYP3A inhibitors and inducers
- Grapefruit juice increases its effects
- Can interact with carbamazepine and similar drugs

Side Effects

- Hair thinning or loss
- GI upset (nausea, diarrhea, mouth sores)

- Fatigue
- Anemia

Nursing Tips

- Monitor liver function and blood counts regularly
- Teach about drug interactions and precautions with food and other medications
- Counsel women on pregnancy prevention during and after therapy

Chapter 15: Medicines for Fluid and Electrolyte Balance

15.1. Drugs and homeostasis

Our bodies rely on a delicate balance—called homeostasis—to keep things like fluid levels and electrolytes in check. But when someone is unwell, this balance can easily be thrown off. Illness isn't the only culprit either; everyday events like losing your appetite, taking certain medications, undergoing surgery, vomiting, or even having diagnostic tests can all disrupt the body's normal fluid and electrolyte levels.

The good news is that there are medications specifically designed to help restore this balance. These drugs work to correct imbalances and support the body's natural ability to maintain a stable internal environment—keeping fluid composition and volume where they should be.

15.2. Electrolyte replacement drugs

Electrolytes are compounds that carry an electric charge when dissolved in water—and they play a vital role in keeping our bodies running smoothly. When someone is ill, or going through certain treatments or physical stresses, these electrolyte levels can drop, disrupting the body's fluid balance. That's where electrolyte replacement drugs come in: they help replenish what's lost and restore the body to its normal state of balance, or homeostasis.

These medications typically contain inorganic or organic salts and are designed to boost deficient electrolytes. Key electrolytes replaced by these drugs include:

- Potassium – the main electrolyte inside our cells (intracellular fluid or ICF)

- Calcium – an important player in the fluid outside cells (extracellular fluid or ECF)
- Magnesium – another crucial electrolyte inside cells, essential for many body functions
- Sodium – the chief ECF electrolyte that's vital for balance and fluid regulation

Potassium: Powering Cells and Muscles

Potassium is the most abundant positively charged ion (cation) in ICF. Since the body doesn't store potassium, we need a consistent intake through food—or if necessary, through medication. When levels are too low, potassium can be replaced orally or intravenously with salts like:

- Potassium acetate
- Potassium chloride
- Potassium gluconate
- Potassium phosphate

Pharmacokinetics

Potassium from oral supplements is easily absorbed through the GI tract. Once it enters the bloodstream, it moves into cells (ICF), aided by an enzyme called adenosine triphosphatase (ATPase), which pumps sodium out and potassium in. The kidneys are the main regulators, excreting excess potassium, with smaller amounts leaving the body through sweat and feces.

Pharmacodynamics

Potassium helps restore depleted levels quickly. It's essential for maintaining the electrical charge of cells and affects how nerves fire and muscles contract—including the heart.

Why Potassium Matters

Potassium is crucial for nerve and muscle function, transmitting impulses, growing and repairing tissue, and keeping acid-base balance in check.

Therapeutic Use

Potassium therapy is used to treat hypokalemia—low potassium in the blood. This can result from:

- Vomiting, diarrhea, nasogastric suction
- Excess urination or kidney issues
- Cystic fibrosis, burns, certain hormone imbalances
- Use of potassium-wasting diuretics, laxative overuse
- Starvation, anorexia, alcoholism, or even clay ingestion
- Use of glucocorticoids, amphotericin B (IV), B12, folic acid, and more

Heart Helper

Potassium can also reduce the toxic effects of digoxin, a heart medication. By stabilizing heart excitability, it helps prevent dangerous arrhythmias associated with digoxin toxicity.

Drug Interactions

Caution is needed when combining potassium with potassium-sparing diuretics (like spironolactone) or ACE inhibitors (like lisinopril), as the risk of hyperkalemia (too much potassium) increases.

Adverse Reactions

Side effects often depend on how the drug is given:

- Oral potassium may cause nausea, vomiting, or diarrhea. Enteric-coated forms can even lead to GI ulcers or blockages.
- IV potassium, if not properly diluted or infused too quickly, may cause pain, vein inflammation, or cardiac arrest. It's especially risky in patients with low urine output.

Nursing Process

Assessment

- Monitor potassium levels, especially if urine output drops
- Watch for signs of hyperkalemia and adverse effects
- Keep an eye on ECG for changes: prolonged PR interval, wide QRS, flat ST segment, tall T waves
- Track intake and output if vomiting or diarrhea is present

Diagnoses

- Risk for fluid imbalance
- Decreased cardiac output
- Knowledge deficit related to therapy

Planning Goals

- Maintain healthy fluid balance
- Avoid arrhythmias
- Ensure proper drug use by patient/caregiver

Implementation

- Use caution with diuretics or ACE inhibitors
- Always dilute IV potassium and infuse slowly—never give as a bolus
- Don't mix potassium phosphate with calcium or magnesium (precipitates form)
- Monitor the IV site for pain or inflammation
- Give oral potassium with meals; treat GI side effects if they arise
- Educate patients and families (see "Teaching about potassium therapy")

Evaluation

- Hydration stays within a healthy range
- Heart rhythm remains stable

- Patient/caregiver understands the medication

Calcium: Strong Bones, Steady Heart

Calcium is a major ECF cation, with 99% stored in bones. When dietary intake is low, the body pulls calcium from bone stores, which can weaken them over time.

Three Forms in the Body

- Bound to proteins like albumin
- Complexed with compounds like phosphate
- Ionized – this form is active and crucial for bodily functions

Calcium Deficiency

Chronic low calcium can cause bone demineralization. Replacement is done orally or via IV with salts like:

- Calcium carbonate
- Calcium chloride
- Calcium citrate
- Calcium gluconate, etc.

Pharmacokinetics

Calcium is absorbed mainly in the upper small intestine, aided by vitamin D, PTH, and an acidic environment. It's stored in bone and mostly excreted in feces.

Pharmacodynamics & Functions

- Essential for nerve and muscle activity
- Supports heart, kidney, and lung function
- Influences blood clotting, membrane stability, and hormonal actions
- Crucial for bone and tooth health

Therapeutic Uses

- Treating magnesium intoxication

- Supporting heart muscle post-resuscitation
- Meeting increased needs during pregnancy, breastfeeding, or childhood
- IV calcium is used for acute hypocalcemia in cases like tetany, alkalosis, or vitamin D deficiency
- Oral calcium helps prevent osteoporosis and treat chronic hypocalcemia due to various conditions

Drug Interactions

- Can worsen digoxin toxicity
- Reduces effect of calcium channel blockers and tetracyclines
- May interact with phosphorus in IV nutrition, risking emboli

Adverse Effects

- Hypercalcemia if unmonitored—causes fatigue, muscle weakness, constipation, and ECG changes
- IV calcium may irritate veins
- IM calcium can cause severe tissue damage

Nursing Process

Assessment

- Monitor calcium levels and ECG for signs of high calcium

Diagnoses

- Cardiac output imbalance
- Risk of injury (e.g., fractures)
- Knowledge deficit

Planning Goals

- Avoid arrhythmias
- Maintain bone strength
- Encourage proper drug use

Implementation

- Infuse IV calcium slowly
- Keep the patient lying down post-injection
- Avoid calcium injections unless absolutely necessary
- Give oral calcium 1–2 hours after meals
- Educate patients on proper use (see "Teaching about calcium therapy")

Evaluation

- Heart stays steady
- Bone health is stable
- Patient and caregivers understand treatment

Magnesium: The Quiet Worker Inside Cells

Magnesium is the second most abundant ICF cation (after potassium) and is essential for enzyme function, nerve transmission, and muscle activity. Most of it is stored in bones and muscles.

Magnesium's Many Roles

- Stimulates PTH to regulate calcium
- Helps with energy production, nerve conduction, and maintaining fluid-electrolyte balance

Causes of Low Magnesium

- Poor absorption or prolonged diarrhea
- Diuretic therapy
- NG suctioning
- Alcohol use
- Medications like cisplatin, aminoglycosides, or amphotericin B

Replacement Options

- IV: magnesium sulfate
- Oral: magnesium oxide

Pharmacokinetics

- Acts quickly when given IV
- Not metabolized; excreted in urine and breast milk

Pharmacodynamics

- Replenishes magnesium stores
- Controls seizures by blocking neuromuscular signals

Therapeutic Use

- Treats symptomatic hypomagnesemia
- Prevents seizures in preeclampsia/eclampsia
- Manages torsades de pointes (a dangerous heart rhythm), and other seizure-related conditions

Drug Interactions

- Can worsen digoxin-induced heart block
- Enhances sedative effects with CNS depressants
- Prolongs action of neuromuscular blockers like succinylcholine

Adverse Effects

- May cause low blood pressure, heart issues, and respiratory paralysis
- IM injections are painful and often repeated

Nursing Process

Assessment

- Monitor intake/output; don't give if urine output is low
- Track ECG and vital signs
- Check serum magnesium and electrolytes

Diagnoses

- Fluid volume imbalance
- Cardiac output disturbance

- Knowledge deficit

Planning Goals

- Maintain fluid balance
- Avoid arrhythmias
- Ensure patient understanding

Implementation

- Always keep calcium gluconate on hand in case of magnesium overdose and respiratory depression

A Knee-Jerk Reaction (Magnesium Monitoring and Administration)

When giving magnesium—especially intravenously—it's essential to monitor the patient closely to avoid serious complications.

- Always check the patient's knee-jerk or patellar reflex before giving each dose. If the reflex is absent, hold the dose and notify the healthcare provider immediately. Skipping this step could result in temporary respiratory failure, which may require CPR or IV calcium to reverse.
- Use extra caution with magnesium in patients who have kidney problems. Impaired kidney function can lead to magnesium building up in the body, increasing the risk of hypermagnesemia (excess magnesium).
- Infuse magnesium sulfate slowly, at a rate no faster than 150 mg per minute. Giving it too fast—especially as a bolus—can be dangerous and may even cause cardiac arrest.
- During infusion, keep a close eye on the patient's vital signs and deep tendon reflexes. Signs of overdose may include low blood pressure and trouble breathing.
- Check serum magnesium levels regularly. After a bolus dose, test the level right after. For patients on continuous IV infusions, monitor magnesium levels at least every 6 hours.

- Patients receiving magnesium replacement should be placed on continuous cardiac monitoring.
- Track urine output closely before, during, and after the infusion. If urine output drops below 100 mL over 4 hours, notify the provider—this may indicate that the body isn't eliminating magnesium effectively.

Evaluation

- The patient stays well-hydrated.
- The patient maintains normal heart function with stable vital signs and ECG.
- The patient and caregivers understand the purpose and safety measures of the drug therapy.

Sodium: A Key Player in Fluid Balance

Sodium is the main cation found in extracellular fluid (ECF), and it plays a big role in keeping things balanced. It helps:

- Maintain osmotic pressure and fluid concentration
- Regulate acid-base and water balance
- Support nerve transmission and muscle function
- Influence glandular secretions

When Sodium Needs a Boost

Sodium replacement becomes necessary in several conditions where sodium levels drop quickly. These include:

- Anorexia, excessive sweating, vomiting, or GI fluid loss
- Overuse of diuretics or tap water enemas
- Trauma, wound drainage, adrenal insufficiency
- Cirrhosis with fluid buildup (ascites)
- SIADH (Syndrome of Inappropriate Antidiuretic Hormone)
- Prolonged IV infusions of plain dextrose (without added electrolytes)

In most cases, sodium is replaced using sodium chloride, either orally or through an IV.

Pharmacokinetics

Sodium chloride, whether taken by mouth or given through an IV, is quickly absorbed and spreads throughout the body. It isn't metabolized much and is excreted mostly in the urine, but also through sweat, tears, and saliva.

Pharmacodynamics

Sodium chloride works by replenishing sodium and chloride ions in the blood, restoring proper fluid and electrolyte balance.

Pharmacotherapeutics

Sodium chloride is used to treat or prevent hyponatremia (low sodium levels) and to restore fluid balance in patients who've lost significant amounts of sodium.

When IV Therapy is Needed

In more severe or symptomatic cases, sodium deficiency is treated through an IV infusion containing sodium chloride.

Drug Interactions

There are no major drug interactions reported with sodium chloride, which makes it relatively straightforward to use.

Adverse Reactions

- Although generally safe when administered properly, sodium can cause problems if infused too rapidly or in large amounts, such as:
- Pulmonary edema (fluid buildup in the lungs)
- Hypernatremia (too much sodium in the blood)
- Potassium loss, which can affect heart rhythm

Nursing Process for Sodium Replacement

Assessment

- Monitor intake and output carefully.
- Check serum electrolyte levels to guide therapy and prevent imbalances.

Key Nursing Diagnoses

- Risk for fluid imbalance due to fluid retention
- Deficient knowledge regarding sodium therapy

Planning Outcome Goals

- The patient maintains appropriate fluid balance based on their age and condition.
- The patient and caregiver understand the purpose and proper use of sodium therapy.

Implementation

- Use sodium cautiously in older adults, postoperative patients, or those with heart failure, kidney issues, circulatory problems, or low protein levels.

Every Breath You Take

Teach patients how to recognize signs of pulmonary edema, such as:

- Shortness of breath
- Coughing
- Anxiety
- Wheezing
- Pale skin

Encourage them to seek medical help immediately if they notice any of these symptoms.

Evaluation

- The patient maintains a normal fluid balance.

- The patient and caregivers can explain the treatment plan and demonstrate understanding of the therapy.

15.3. Alkalinizing and Acidifying Drugs

Alkalinizing and Acidifying Drugs

When the body's acid-base balance is off, it can affect everything from breathing to heart function. That's where alkalinizing and acidifying drugs come in. These medications help bring blood pH levels back to a healthy range—either by neutralizing excess acid or by making the blood more acidic when it's too alkaline.

Opposites That Work Together

Although these drugs do opposite things, they share the same goal: restoring balance.

- Alkalinizing drugs raise the pH of the blood by decreasing hydrogen ion concentration.
- Acidifying drugs lower the pH by increasing hydrogen ion concentration.

Interestingly, some of these drugs also affect urine pH, which can be helpful for managing certain urinary tract infections or even treating drug overdoses.

Alkalinizing Drugs

These are used primarily to treat metabolic acidosis, a condition where there's too much acid (hydrogen ions) in the blood, leading to a lower-than-normal pH.

Common alkalinizing drugs include:

- Sodium bicarbonate (also used to alkalinize urine)
- Sodium citrate
- Sodium lactate
- Tromethamine (THAM)

How They Work (Pharmacokinetics)

- These drugs are well absorbed orally.
- Sodium bicarbonate isn't metabolized—it acts directly.
- Sodium citrate and sodium lactate are converted into bicarbonate, the body's natural buffer.
- Tromethamine is largely excreted unchanged in the urine.

What They Do (Pharmacodynamics)

- Sodium bicarbonate works by releasing bicarbonate ions into the bloodstream, which neutralize excess hydrogen ions and raise blood pH. As it gets excreted in urine, the urine pH also increases.
- Sodium citrate and sodium lactate act similarly after being converted to bicarbonate.
- Tromethamine binds directly with hydrogen ions to help reduce acidity, and the complex is then eliminated through urine.

When They're Used (Pharmacotherapeutics)

Alkalinizing drugs are used to:

- Treat metabolic acidosis
- Alkalinize urine to help clear substances like phenobarbital in overdose cases

Drug Interactions

These medications may interfere with other drugs:

- Reduce the effects of: ketoconazole, lithium, salicylates
- Increase the effects of: amphetamines, pseudoephedrine, quinidine
- Reduce antibacterial activity of methenamine

Tromethamine has no significant drug interactions.

Side Effects to Watch For

Each drug has its own potential adverse effects:

- Sodium bicarbonate: Overuse can lead to metabolic alkalosis. Rapid IV infusion, especially in diabetic ketoacidosis, can cause brain dysfunction, oxygen issues, and lactic acidosis. Its sodium content can lead to fluid retention and edema. Orally, it may cause bloating or gas.
- Sodium citrate: Overdose may cause alkalosis or tetany and worsen heart conditions. It can also act as a laxative.
- Sodium lactate: Similar to bicarbonate and citrate, it can cause metabolic alkalosis. Watch for fluid overload in patients with kidney or heart issues.
- Tromethamine: May cause injection site irritation (like phlebitis), and more serious effects like low blood sugar, respiratory depression, or high potassium. Prolonged use (over 24 hours) can result in toxicity.

Nursing Process: Alkalinizing Drugs

Assessment

- Monitor pH and bicarbonate levels
- Watch for signs of overdose: irritability, twitching, tetany
- Track fluid input/output
- Be alert to drug interactions and side effects
- Check patient and caregiver knowledge

Diagnoses

- Risk of injury due to drug effects
- Knowledge gap about therapy

Planning Goals

- Prevent injury from side effects
- Patient/caregiver will understand drug use

Implementation

- Monitor IV sites closely—especially for sodium bicarbonate, sodium lactate, and tromethamine

457

- If extravasation happens, elevate the limb, apply warm compresses, and consider using lidocaine
- Don't use tromethamine longer than 24 hours
- Educate patients and caregivers on what to watch for

Evaluation

- Patient avoids injury or complications
- Patient and caregiver show understanding of therapy

Acidifying Drugs

These are used to correct metabolic alkalosis, which happens when there's too much bicarbonate or not enough acid in the body—raising blood pH too high.

Common acidifying drugs include:

- Acetazolamide (also used for altitude sickness and glaucoma)
- Ammonium chloride
- Ascorbic acid (vitamin C) – used mainly to acidify urine

How They Work (Pharmacokinetics)

- Acetazolamide starts working quickly by blocking carbonic anhydrase, an enzyme that helps the kidneys excrete acid. This leads to more bicarbonate being excreted, reducing pH.
- Ammonium chloride is absorbed in 3–6 hours and converted by the liver into urea and hydrochloric acid, which then lowers blood pH.
- Ascorbic acid is absorbed well when taken orally, metabolized in the liver, and excreted in urine.

What They Do (Pharmacodynamics)

- Acetazolamide: Increases bicarbonate excretion → lowers blood pH
- Ammonium chloride: Becomes hydrochloric acid in the body → adds hydrogen ions → lowers blood/urine pH

- Ascorbic acid: Directly releases hydrogen ions into urine, lowering urine pH

When They're Used (Pharmacotherapeutics)

- Used to correct metabolic alkalosis
- Often, patients receive both hydrogen ions and chloride ions (as in ammonium chloride) for safe and effective therapy

Note: Acetazolamide might not work well in patients with kidney issues and can lead to potassium loss.

Drug Interactions

- Generally minimal, but combining ammonium chloride with spironolactone may increase the risk of systemic acidosis

Side Effects to Watch For

- Acetazolamide: Nausea, vomiting, hypokalemia, drowsiness, altered taste, and in rare cases, aplastic anemia
- Ammonium chloride: May lead to metabolic acidosis, especially in high doses. Can also cause loss of electrolytes like potassium
- Ascorbic acid: High doses can irritate the GI tract and, in patients with G6PD deficiency, may cause hemolytic anemia

Nursing Process: Acidifying Drugs

Assessment

- Monitor blood pH, bicarbonate, and potassium levels
- Look for signs of acidosis or low potassium
- In patients with G6PD deficiency, monitor complete blood count for anemia
- Review patient and caregiver understanding of therapy

Diagnoses

- Fluid volume imbalance due to fluid shifts
- Injury risk from side effects

- Knowledge deficit

Planning Goals

- Patient avoids fluid overload
- Injury risk is minimized
- Patient and caregiver understand the therapy

Implementation

- Administer IV acidifying drugs slowly to avoid local pain and systemic effects
- If hypokalemia develops, notify the provider and correct it
- Instruct patients to report GI side effects or signs of worsening symptoms
- For ascorbic acid or ammonium chloride, monitor urine pH and report any serious side effects
- Twitching during ammonium chloride therapy could signal toxicity—hold the next dose and contact the provider
- If headaches or insomnia occur, offer comfort measures or seek treatment (like a mild analgesic or hypnotic)

Evaluation

- Patient maintains healthy fluid balance
- No injuries from side effects occur
- Patient and caregivers can explain and manage the treatment plan

Printed in Dunstable, United Kingdom

71825898R00261